MEDICAL
ACRONYMS,
EPONYMS &
ABBREVIATIONS

THIRD EDITION

Marilyn Fuller Delong, RN, BSN, MA

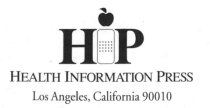

HIP

HEALTH INFORMATION PRESS

Los Angeles, California 90010

Delong, Marilyn Fuller
    Medical acronyms, eponyms & abbreviations / by
Marilyn Fuller Delong. -- 3rd ed.
        p.   cm.
    ISBN 1-57066-007-7
    1. Medicine--Abbreviations. 2. Medicine--Acronyms.
3. Medicine--Eponyms. I. Title. II. Title: Medical
acronyms, eponyms and abbreviations
    [DNLM: 1. Medicine--abbreviations. 2. Medicine--
acronyms. 3. Medicine--Eponyms. W13 D361m 1994]
R123.D455 1997
610'.148--dc20
DNLM/DLC
for Library of Congress   94-40393
                                              CIP

ISBN 1-885987-05-6

Health Information Press
A division of Practice Management Information Corp. (PMIC)
4727 Wilshire Blvd., Suite 300
Los Angeles, CA 90010
1-800-MED-SHOP

http://medicalbookstore.com

Printed in the United States of America

This publication is designed to offer basic information regarding medical acronyms, abbreviations and eponyms. The information presented is based on the experience and interpretation of the author. Though all of the information has been carefully researched and checked for accuracy, neither the author nor the publisher accept any responsibility or liability with regard to errors, omissions, misuse or misinterpretation.

About the Author

Marilyn Fuller Delong, RN, BSN, is a nurse consultant and writer specializing in utilization review, discharge planning and case management. Her professional experience has included ICU, CCU and ER nursing in Iowa, Texas as well as California. She has been an instructor at St. Luke's School of Nursing in Cedar Rapids, Iowa; associate editor of the Journal of Quality Assurance; and a contributor to several health-related publications. She is a member of state and national associations of quality assurance professionals.

Dedication

Dedicated to the loving memory of my father, Robert J. Fuller

Table of Contents

Eponyms

Introduction

To the lay person, medical documents are intimidating, and for good reason.

Not only are they filled with lots of Latin terms and phrases, but they also contain an endless assortment of abbreviations. Supposedly these stand for something important, but what?

Medical Acronyms, Eponyms and Abbreviations is designed to help you answer that question. It translates those seemingly meaningless letters into something meaningful.

Nearly all medical personnel who enter information on a patient's chart write in cryptic symbols. Even medical journals and textbooks rely extensively on such conventions. Deciphering this jargon is vitally important, whether you are a patient taking control of your own healthcare, or a health science student taking a test.

Take for example **A.K.A.**, which many people would read as "also known as." Its predominant medical meaning is "above the knee amputation."

And many abbreviations have more than one meaning. For example, **B.S.** can mean Bachelor of Science, or barium swallow (an x-ray), or blood sugar, or bowel sounds, or Blue Shield. Without a comprehensive list of the possible definitions, as you will find in this book, an inappropriate connotation might be assigned to a term.

Acronyms are words that are formed from the initial letter or letters of words in a phrase. You might already know from television that **MASH** stands for **M**obile **A**rmy **S**urgical **H**ospital. From this book, you will also learn that a **BRAT** is a diet of **b**ananans, **r**ice cereal, **a**pples and **t**oast; that **MOM** is **m**ilk **of m**agnesia; and that **PET** means **p**ositron **e**mission **t**omography.

Eponyms use the name of a person to describe a disease or other phenomenon. It is certainly an honor for the named person, but less descriptive for the medical reader. **Hansen disease** just doesn't have the same impact as leprosy, and **VonWillebrand disease** doesn't carry the connotation of hemophilia. The book translates these and other eponyms into their more descriptive medical terms.

Who should use this book? Anyone who needs to accurately decode and interpret medical records and information.

Of course this includes health care workers, medical transcriptionists, and students. This book can even be used by fiction writers who want to add realism to their stories of hospital intrigue and physician romance.

But in today's changing health environment, it is increasingly important for patients to know exactly what their doctors are diagnosing; to know what treatments are being prescribed; and to know what their medical insurance is being billed.

The most difficult part in compiling entries for this book was in stopping. New acronyms, eponyms and abbreviations are created every day. Hopefully this will answer the vast majority of information needs you have.

SYMBOLS

General Symbols

↓		decrease
↑		increase
○	♀	female
□	♂	male
*		birth
†		death
∞		infinity
1°		primary
2°		secondary
2-D		two dimensional
3-D		three dimensional

Apothecary Symbols

ī	one
ī/d	once a day
īī	two
īīī	three
s̄s̄	one-half
ʒ	dram
℥	ounce
ʒi	one teaspoon
℥i	one ounce

℩   minim

Greek Letters

α   lower-case alpha; alpha particle; Bunsen's solubility
           coefficient; prefix denoting first of a series

αCD   alpha-chain disease

β   lower-case beta; beta particle; buffer capacity; prefix
           denoting second of a series

β2m   beta$_2$ microglobulin

γ   lower-case gamma; gamma ray or other photon;
           microgram; prefix denoting third of a series

δ   lower-case delta; prefix denoting fourth of a series

Δ   upper-case delta; amount of change or difference; prism
           diopter

ε   lower-case epsilon; dielectric constant; molar
           absorptivity; permitivity

η   lower-case eta; absolute viscosity (Poiseuille's viscosity
           coefficient)

Θ   upper-case theta; kinetic constant

λ   lower-case lambda; microliter; Ostwald's solubility
           coefficient; radioactive decay constant; wavelength

μ   lower-case mu; dipole moment, magnetic moment;
           dynamic viscosity; micro-; micrometer (micron);
           permeability; statistical mean

μg   microgamma

μμ   micromicro-; micromicron

μμg   micromicrogram (picogram)

μW   microhm

μA   microampere

μc   microcurie

μC   microcoulomb

μCi	microcurie
μEq	milliequivalent
μF	microfarad
μg	microgram
μIU	micro-international unit
μl	microliter
μL	microliter
μm	micrometer (micron)
μmol	micromole (micromol)
μN	micronormal
μOsm	micro-osmole (micro-osmol)
μs	microsecond
μsec	microsecond
μU	microunit
μV	microvolt
μW	microwatt
ν	lower-case nu; frequency; kinematic viscosity
π	lower-case pi; osmotic pressure; ratio of circumference of a circle to its diameter
Π	upper-case pi; product of (by multiplication)
ρ	lower-case rho; electric charge density; mass density (g/cm^3); population correlation coefficient
σ	lower-case sigma; reflection coefficient; standard deviation; surface tension; wave number
$σ^2$	variance for a normal distribution
σD	standard deviation of the difference
Σ	upper-case sigma; sum of

Σ_{ST}	total depression or elevation of ST segments in all ECG leads
τ	lower-case tau; life (time); mean life; relaxation time
$\tau^1/_2$	half-life
ϕ	lower-case phi; osmotic coefficient; phenyl-
Φ	upper-case phi; magnetic flux
χ	lower-case chi; susceptibility (electric, magnetic)
χ^2	chi-square, a test of statistical significance
ψ	lower-case psi; wave function
Ω	upper-case omega; ohm (unit of electrical resistance)

A

a	accommodation • acid, acidity • alpha • ampere • anode • anterior • area • artery, arterial • asymmetric • at • axial • before *(ante)* • water *(aqua)*
ā	before *(ante)*
A	abnormal • absorbance • adenine • adenosine • adult • age • allergy • alpha • alternate • alveolar • ampere • Angstrom unit • anterior • area • atropine • axial • axillary (temperature) • symbol for mass number • water *(aqua)* • year *(annus)*
A₂	aortic second sound
āā	of each *(ana)*
A-a	alveolar-arterial (gradient)
AA	achievement age • Alcoholics Anonymous • amino acid • anticipatory avoidance • aplastic anemia • arteries • Associate in Arts (degree) • atomic absorption (spectrophotometer) • author's alteration • automobile accident.
aaa	amalgam
AAA	abdominal aortic aneurysm • acquired aplastic anemia • acute anxiety attack • addiction, autoimmune diseases, and aging • American Academy of Allergy • American Academy of Anatomists • American Allergy Association • androgenic anabolic agent
AAAAA	aphasia, agnosia, apraxia, agraphia, alexia
AAAHC	American Association for Ambulatory Health Care
AAAI	American Academy of Allergy and Immunology
AAAS	American Association for the Advancement of Science

AABB	American Association of Blood Banks
AAC	antibiotic-associated colitis
AACCN	American Association of Critical Care Nurses
AACHP	American Association for Comprehensive Health Planning
AACIA	American Association for Clinical Immunology and Allergy
AACN	American Association of Critical-Care Nurses • American Association of Colleges of Nursing
AAD	American Academy of Dermatology
AADS	American Academy of Dental Schools
A-aDO$_2$	alveolar-arterial oxygen difference (gradient)
AAE	active assistive exercise • acute allergic encephalitis • Affirmative Action Employer • American Association of Endodontists
AAF	acetic-alcohol-formalin (fixing fluid) • acetylaminofluorene • ascorbic acid factor
AAFA	Asthma and Allergy Foundation of America
AAFP	American Academy of Family Physicians • American Academy of Family Practice
AAGP	American Academy of General Practice
AAHA	American Association for Homes for the Aging
AAHPERD	American Alliance for Health, Physical Education, Recreation and Dance
AAI	American Association of Immunologists
AAIN	American Association of Industrial Nurses
AAL	anterior axillary line
AAMA	American Association of Medical Assistants
AAMC	American Association of Medical Colleges
AAMD	American Association on Mental Deficiency
AAME	acetylargenine methyl ester
AAMRL	American Association of Medical Records Librarians

AAMS	acute aseptic meningitis syndrome
AAMSI	American Association for Medical Systems and Informatics
AAN	American Academy of Neurology • American Academy of Nursing • amino acid nitrogen
AANA	American Anorexia Nervosa Association • American Association of Nurse-Anesthetists
AANN	American Association of Neuroscience Nurses
AANS	American Academy of Neurological Surgery • American Association of Neurological Surgeons
AAO	American Academy of Ophthalmology • American Academy of Otolaryngology • American Association of Orthodontists • American Association of Osteopathy
AAOG	American Association of Obstetricians and Gynecologists
AAOO	American Academy of Ophthalmology and Otolaryngology
AAOP	American Academy of Oral Pathology
AAOS	American Academy of Orthopaedic Surgeons
AAP	air at atmospheric pressure • American Academy of Pediatrics • American Association of Pathologists
AAPA	American Academy of Physician Assistants
AAPB	American Association of Pathologists and Bacteriologists
AAPC	annual average per capita
A-a pCO$_2$	alveolar-arterial pCO$_2$ (gradient)
AAPMR	American Academy of Physical Medicine and Rehabilitation
AAR	Australia antigen radioimmunoassay
AARC	American Association for Respiratory Care
AAROM	active assist range of motion
AARP	American Association of Retired Persons

AAS	acute abdominal series • anthrax antiserum • aortic arch syndrome • atomic absorption spectrophotometry
AASEC	American Association of Sex Educators and Counselors
AAT	acute abdominal tympany • alpha-1 antitrypsin
AAU	acute anterior uveitis
AAV	adeno-associated virus
ab	abortion, abort • about
Ab	abortion, antibody, antibodies
AB	abortion • Aid to the Blind • alcian blue • antibiotic • apex beat • asthmatic bronchitis • axiobuccal • Bachelor of Arts (*Artium Baccalaureus*)
A/B	acid-base ratio
A&B	apnea and bradycardia
ABA	abscisic acid • American Board of Anesthesiology
ABAI	American Board of Allergy and Immunology
AbAP	antibody-against-panel
ABBS	American Brittle Bone Society
ABC	airway, breathing, circulation • antigen-binding capacity • apnea, bradycardia, cyanosis • applesauce, bananas, cereal (diet) aspiration biopsy cytology • atomic, biological, chemical • axiobuccocervical
ABC&C&C	airway, breathing, circulation, cervical spine, consciousness level
ABCRS	American Board of Colon and Rectal Surgery
abd	abdomen, abdominal • abduction, abductor
ABD	American Board of Dermatology
abdom	abdomen, abdominal
ABE	acute bacterial endocarditis • trivalent antitoxin for types A, B, and E botulism

ABEM	American Board of Emergency Medicine
ABFP	American Board of Family Practice
ABG	arterial blood gases • axiobuccogingival
ABIM	American Board of Internal Medicine
ABL	a-beta-lipoproteinemia • antigen-binding lymphocytes • axiobuccolingual
ABLB	alternate binaural loudness balance (test)
ABMS	American Board of Medical Specialties
abn	abnormal
ABNM	American Board of Nuclear Medicine
abnorm	abnormal
ABNS	American Board of Neurological Surgery
ABO	absent bed occupant • American Board of Ophthalmology • American Board of Otolaryngology • major blood group system
ABOG	American Board of Obstetrics and Gynecology
ABOS	American Board of Orthopaedic Surgery
ABP	Adriamycin, bleomycin, prednisone • androgen-binding protein • arterial blood pressure
ABPA	acute bronchopulmonary asthma
ABPM	American Board of Preventive Medicine
ABPMR	American Board of Physical Medicine and Rehabilitation
ABPN	American Board of Psychiatry and Neurology
ABPS	American Board of Plastic Surgery
ABR	absolute bed rest • American Board of Radiology • auditory brain-stem response
abras	abrasion
abs	absent, absence • absolute • absorbance
ABS	acute brain syndrome • American Board of Surgery
absc	abscissa

abs feb	in the absence of fever *(absente febre)*
absorb	absorption
abstr	abstract
ABT	autologous bone marrow transplantation
ABTS	American Board of Thoracic Surgery
ABU	American Board of Urology
ABVD	Adriamycin, bleomycin, vinblastine, dacarbazine
abx	antibiotics
ABY	acid bismuth yeast agar
ac	acetyl • acute • alternating current • before meals *(ante cibum)* • assisted control
Ac	actinium
AC	acetylcholine • acetylcysteine • acid • acromioclavicular • acute • adherent cell • admission certification • adrenal cortex • Adriamycin, cyclophosphamide • air conduction • alternating current • anodal closure • anterior chamber • anticoagulant • anti-inflammatory corticoid • aortic closure • atriocarotid • auriculocarotid • axiocervical
A/C	albumin-coagulin ratio
ACA	adenocarcinoma • American College of Anesthesiologists • aminocaproic acid • anterior cerebral artery • Automatic Clinical Analyzer
acad	academy
ACB	American Council of the Blind • aortocoronary (saphenous vein) bypass • arterialized capillary blood
acc	acceleration • accident • accommodation • according
ACC	adenoid cystic carcinoma • alveolar-cell carcinoma • ambulatory care center • American College of Cardiology • American College of Cryosurgery • anodal closure contraction • aplasia cutis congenita
accel	acceleration

AcCh	acetylcholine
ACCl	anodal closure clonus
accid	accident
AcCoA	acetylcoenzyme A
accom	accommodation
ACCP	American College of Chest Physicians
accum	accumulation
ACD	absolute cardiac dullness • acid-citrate-dextrose (solution) • anterior chest diameter • area of cardiac disease
ACDF	anterior cervical discectomy and fusion
ACE	acute care of the elderly • adrenal cortical (adrenocortical) extract • aerobic chair exercises • angiotensin-converting enzyme
ACEP	American College of Emergency Physicians
ACF	accessory clinical findings
ac-G	accelerator globulin
ACG	American College of Gastroenterology • angiocardiogram, angiocardiography • apexcardiogram, apexcardiography
ACGME	Accreditation Council for Graduate Medical Education
ACh	acetylcholine
ACH	adrenal cortical (adrenocortical) hormone • arm, chest, height
ACHA	American College of Hospital Administrators
AChE	acetylcholinesterase
AChR	acetylcholine receptor
ACI	after-care instructions • anticlonus index
ACIDS	acquired cellular immunodeficient syndrome
ACIP	Advisory Committee on Immunization Practices
ACL	anterior cruciate ligament

ACLA	American Clinical Laboratory Association
ACLS	advance cardiac life support
ACN	acute conditioned necrosis
ACNM	American College of Nurse-Midwives
ACNP	American College of Neuropsychopharmacology
ACOG	American College of Obstetricians and Gynecologists
ACOMS	American College of Oral and Maxillofacial Surgeons
ACOS	American College of Osteopathic Surgeons
ACP	acyl-carrier protein • American College of Pathologists • American College of Physicians • aspirin, caffeine, phenacetin • Association of Clinical Pathologists
ac phos	acid phosphatase
ACPM	American College of Preventive Medicine
ACPP	adrenocorticopolypeptide
ACPPD	average cost per patient day
ACPS	acrocephalopolysyndactyly
ACR	American College of Radiology • anticonstipation regimen
ACS	acute confusional state • ambulatory care services • American Cancer Society • American Celiac Society • American College of Surgeons • anodal closing sound • antireticular cytotoxic serum • aperture current setting
ACSM	American College of Sports Medicine
ACSW	Academy of Certified Social Workers
act	active, activity
ACT	achievement through counseling and treatment • activated clotting time • activated coagulation time • anticoagulant therapy • asthma care training
ACTD	actinomycin D
ACTe	anodal closure tetanus

ACTH	adrenocorticotropic hormone
activ	activity
ACTN	adrenocorticotrophin
ACTP	adrenocorticotropic polypeptide
ACU	acute care unit • ambulatory care unit
ACV	assist control ventilation
ACVD	acute cardiovascular disease
AC/W	acetone in water
ad	let there be added *(adde)* • to, toward, up to *(ad)*
AD	achievement drive • addicted to drugs • admitting diagnosis • advanced directive • after discharge • alcohol dehydrogenase • Alzheimer's disease • adenoidal degeneration • anodal duration • autosomal dominant • average deviation • right atrium *(atrium dextrum)* • right ear *(auris dextra)* • axiodistal
ADA	American Dental Association • American Diabetes Association • American Dietetic Association • Americans with Disabilities Act
ADAA	American Dental Assistants Association
ADAMHA	Alcohol, Drug Abuse and Mental Health Administration
AdC	adrenal cortex
ADC	Aid to Dependent Children • albumin, dextrose, catalase • anodal duration contraction • average daily census • axiodistalcervical
ADCC	antibody-dependent cellular cytotoxicity
add	adduction, adductor • let there be added *(adde)*
ADD	attention deficit disorder
ad def an	to the point of fainting *(ad defectionem animi)*
ADE	acute disseminated encephalitis
ADEA	Age Discrimination in Employment Act
ADEM	acute disseminated encephalomyelitis

adeq	adequate
ADG	axiodistogingival
ADH	adhesions • alcohol dehydrogenase • antidiuretic hormone
ADHA	American Dental Hygienists Association
adhib	to be administered *(adhibendus)*
ADI	acceptable daily intake • axiodistoincisal
adj	adjunct
ADL	activities of daily life, activities of daily living
ad lib	freely, as desired *(ad libitum)*
adm	administrator, administration • admit, admission
AdM	adrenal medulla
ADM	administrative medicine • adriamycin
ADME	absorption, distribution, metabolism, excretion
admov	apply, let it be applied *(admove, admoveatur)*
ADN	Associate Degree in Nursing
ADO	axiodisto-occlusal
ADP	adenosine diphosphate • area diastolic pressure • automated data processing
ADPL	average daily patient load
ADR	Acceptable Dental Remedies • actual death rate • adverse drug reaction
ADRN	Associate Degree Registered Nurse
ADS	antibody deficient syndrome • antidiuretic substance
adst feb	while fever is present *(adstante febre)*
ADT	adenosine triphosphate • admission, discharge, transfer • agar-gel diffusion test • alternate day treatment • automated dithionite test • placebo ("Any Desired Thing")
ADTe	anodal duration tetanus
adv	against *(adversum)*

A-DV	arterial-deep venous difference
advert	advertisement
ADX	adrenalectomized
AE	above elbow • acrodermatitis enteropathica • activation energy
A/E	above elbow
AEA	alcohol, ether, acetone
AEC	at earliest convenience • Atomic Energy Commission
AED	automatic external defibrillator
aeg	the patient *(aeger, aegra)*
AEG	air encephalogram
AEL	acute erythroleukemia
AEM	analytical electron microscope
AEP	admission evaluation protocol • auditory evoked potential • average evoked potential
aer	aerosol
AER	acoustic evoked response • albumin excretion rate • aldosterone excretion rate • auditory evoked response • average evoked response
AES	antieosinophilic sera
aet	at the age of, aged *(aetas)*
aetat	of age *(aetatis)*
AEV	avian erythroblastosis virus
AEVS	automated eligibility verification system
af	audiofrequency
AF	acid-fast • albumin free (tuberculin) • amniotic fluid • aortic flow • aortofemoral • Arthritis Foundation • atrial fibrillation • atrial flutter • audio frequency • auricular fibrillation
AFA	alcohol-formalin-acetic acid (solution)

AFB	acid-fast bacillus • American Foundation for the Blind
AFB₁	aflatoxin B1
AFCR	American Federation for Clinical Research
AFDC	Aid to Families with Dependent Children
aff	afferent
AFH	adenofibromatous hyperplasia • anterior facial height
AFI	amaurotic familiar idiocy
AFib	atrial fibrillation
AFIP	Armed Forces Institute of Pathology
AFMS	Affective Family Member Syndrome
AFO	ankle-foot orthosis (splint)
AFP	alpha-fetoprotein
AFR	ascorbic free radical
AFRD	acute febrile respiratory disease
AFRI	acute febrile respiratory illness
AFS	American Fertility Society
AFTC	apparent free testosterone concentration
AFX	atypical fibroxanthoma
ag	atrial gallop
Ag	antigen • silver *(argentum)*
AG	aminoglutethimide • antiglobulin • antigravity • atrial gallop • axiogingival
A/G	albumin-globulin ratio
AGA	accelerated growth area • American Gastroenterological Association • American Geriatrics Association • appropriate for gestational age
AgCl	silver chloride
AGD	agar gel diffusion
AGE	acute gastroenteritis • angle of greatest extension

AGF	angle of greatest flexion
agg	agglutinate, agglutination
AGG	agammaglobulinemia
aggl	agglutinate, agglutination
aggreg	aggregation
AGGS	anti-gas gangrene serum
agit	shake *(agita)*
agit bene	shake well *(agita bene)*
agit vas	the vial being shaken *(agitato vase)*
AGL	acute granulocytic leukemia
AGMK	African green monkey kidney
AGN	acute glomerulonephritis • agnosia
AgNO$_3$	silver nitrate
AGOS	American Gynecological and Obstetrical Society
AGPA	American Group Practice Association
AGS	adrenogenital syndrome • American Geriatrics Society
agt	agent
AGT	antiglobulin test • adrenoglomerulotrophin
AGTT	abnormal glucose tolerance test
AGV	aniline gentian violet
AH	abdominal hysterectomy • amenorrhea and hirsutism • antihyaluronidase • arterial hypertension • hypermetropic astigmatism
A&H	accident and health insurance
AHA	acquired hemolytic anemia • American Heart Association • American Hospital Association • autoimmune hemolytic anemia
AHC	acute hemorrhagic conjunctivitis • acute hemorrhagic cystitis

AHCPR	Agency for Health Care Policy and Research (of the Dept. of Health and Human Services)
AHD	antihypertensive drug • arteriosclerotic heart disease • atherosclerotic heart disease • autoimmune hemolytic disease
AHE	acute hemorrhagic encephalomyelitis
AHEC	area health-education center
AHF	antihemolytic factor • antihemophilic factor
AHFS	American Hospital Formulary Service
AHFS-DI	American Hospital Formulary Service-Drug Information
AHG	antihemophilic globulin • antihuman globulin
AHGS	acute herpetic gingival stomatitis
AHH	arylhydrocarbon hydroxylase
AHIMA	American Health Information Management Association
AHIP	assisted health insurance plan
AHN	Assistant Head Nurse
AHP	acute hemorrhagic pancreatitis • allied health professionals
AHR	autonomic hyperreflexia
AHTG	antihuman thymocytic globulin
AHTP	antihuman thymocytic plasma
AI	accidentally incurred • aortic insufficiency • apical impulse • artificial insemination • artificial intelligence • atherogenic index • atrial insufficiency • axioincisal
AIB	aminoisobutyric acid
AIBA	aminoisobutyric acid
AIBS	American Institute of Biological Sciences
AICAR	aminoimidazole carboxamide ribonucleotide
AICD	Automatic Implantable Cardioverter Defibrillator

AICF	autoimmune complement fixation
AID	acute infectious disease • Agency for International Development • artificial insemination donor
AIDS	acquired immune deficiency syndrome
AIE	acute infective endocarditis
AIF	aortic-iliac-femoral
AIG	anti-immunoglobulin
AIH	artificial insemination, homologous
AIHA	autoimmune hemolytic anemia
AIHD	acquired immune hemolytic disease
AIL	angioimmunoblastic lymphadenopathy
AILC	adult independent living center
AILD	angioimmunoblastic lymphadenopathy with dysproteinemia
AIM	artificial intelligence in medicine
AIMS	abnormal involuntary movement scale
AIP	acute idiopathic pericarditis • acute inflammatory polyneuropathy • acute intermittent porphyria • annual implementation plan • average intravascular pressure
AIS	androgen insensitivity syndrome
AIT	administrator-in-training
AIU	absolute iodine uptake
AIUM	American Institute of Ultrasound in Medicine
AIVR	accelerated idioventricular rhythm
AJ	ankle jerk
AJC	American Joint Commission (Study for Cancer Staging and End Results Reporting)
AJN	American Journal of Nursing
AK	above knee
AKA	above-knee amputation • also known as

AK amp	above-knee amputation
AKBR	arterial ketone body ratio
AKV	acrokeratosis verruciformis
Al	aluminum
AL	adaptation level • alignment mark • arterial line • axiolingual
Ala	alanine
ALa	axiolabial
ALA	American Lung Association • aminolevulinic acid
ALA-D	aminolevulinic acid dehydrase
ALaG	axiolabiogingival
alb	albumin • white *(albus)*
alc	alcohol, alcoholism
ALC	alternative level of care • avian leukosis complex • axiolinguocervical
Alc R	alcohol rub
ALD	adrenoleukodystrophy • alcoholic liver disease • aldolase
ALE	allowable limits of error
alg	algebraic
ALG	antilymphocytic globulin • axiolinguogingival
ALH	anterior lobe hormone • anterior lobe of hypophysis
A-line	arterial line
ALJ	administrative law judge
alk	alkaline
alk agents	alkylating agents
alk phos	alkaline phosphatase
alk p'tase	alkaline phosphatase
all	allergy

ALL	acute lymphatic leukemia • acute lymphoblastic leukemia • acute lymphocytic leukemia
ALLO	atypical legionnaires-like organism
ALMI	anterolateral myocardial infarction
ALMV	anterior leaflet of mitral valve
ALN	anterior lymph node
ALO	axiolinguo-occlusal
ALOH	average length of hospitalization
ALOS	average length of stay
ALP	acute lupus pericarditis • alkaline phosphatase • anterior lobe of pituitary
ALROS	American Laryngological, Rhinological, and Otological Society
ALS	advanced life support • amyotropic lateral sclerosis • antilymphocytic serum
alt	alternate • altitude
ALT	alanine (amino) transaminase
ALT/AST	ratio of serum alanine aminotransferase to serum aspartate aminotransferase
ALTB	acute laryngotracheobronchitis
alt dieb	every other day *(alternis diebus)*
alt hor	every other hour *(alternis horis)*
alt noc	every other night *(alternis noctus)*
alv	alveolar
ALW	arch-loop-whorl (system)
am	ametropia • amyl • before noon *(ante meridiem)* • meter-angle • myopic astigmatism
Am	americium

AM	actomyosin • ambulatory • amethopterin • ampere meter • amplitude modulation • anovular menstruation • arousal mechanism • aviation medicine • axiomesial • before noon (*ante meridien*) myopic astigmatism
AMA	against medical advice • American Medical Association • antimitochondrial antibody
AMA-DE	American Medical Association-Drug Evaluations
amb	ambient • ambiguous • ambulance • ambulatory
AMC	academic medical center • arthrogryposis multiplex congenita • axiomesiocervical
AMCHA	aminomethylcyclohexane- carboxylic acid
AMEEGA	American Medical Electroencephalographic Association
AMEL	Aero-Medical Equipment Laboratory
Amer	American
AMEND	Aiding Mothers Experiencing Neonatal Death
AMESLAN	American Sign Language
AMG	axiomesiogingival
AMH	Accreditation Manual for Hospitals • automated medical history • mixed astigmatism with myopia predominating
AMHT	automated multiphasic health testing
AMI	acute myocardial infarction • amitryptline • anterior myocardial infarction • axiomesioincisal
AML	acanthiomeatal line • acute myeloblastic leukemia • acute myelogenous leukemia • acute myeloid leukemia • acute myelomonocytic leukemia • automated Medicare log
Am Lev	aminolevulinic acid
AMM	agnogenic myeloid metaplasia
ammon	ammonia
AMol	acute monoblastic leukemia • acute monocytic leukemia

AMO	axiomesio-occlusal
AMOL	acute monocytic leukemia
amor	amorphous
amp	ampere • amplification • ampule • amputate, amputation
AMP	accelerated mental process • adenosine monophosphate (adenylate, adenylic acid) • amphetamine • ampicillin • average mean pressure
AMPAC	American Medical Political Action Committee
amp-hr	ampere-hour
AMPS	acid mucopolysaccharide
AMPT	alpha-methylparatyrosine
AMR	alternate motion rate
AMRS	automated Medical-record system
AMS	altered mental status • auditory memory span • automated multiphasic screening
amt	amount
AMT	American Medical Technologists
amu	atomic mass unit
AMV	avian myeloblastosis virus
AMVI	acute mesenteric vascular insufficiency
AMVL	anterior mitral valve leaflet
AMWA	American Medical Women's Association • American Medical Writers' Association
An	actinon • anisometropia • anode, anodal • antigen
A$_n$	normal atmosphere
AN	acne neonatorum • anesthesia services • anorexia nervosa • anterior • avascular necrosis
ana	each (*ana*)
ANA	American Neurological Association • American Nurses' Association • antinuclear antibody

ANAD	anorexia nervosa and associated disorders • National Association of Anorexia Nervosa and Associated Disorders
anal	analgesic • analysis, analyst, analytic, analyze
ANAP	agglutination negative, absorption positive
anat	anatomy, anatomical
ANC	acid-neutralizing capacity • Army Nurse Corps
AnCC	anodal closure contraction
ANCC	anodal closure contraction
AND	administratively necessary days • anterior nasal discharge
ANDA	Abbreviated New Drug Application
ANDTe	anodal duration tetanus
anes	anesthesia, anesthesiology
anesth	anesthesia, anesthesiology
an ex	anode excitation
ANF	American Nurses' Federation • American Nurses' Foundation • antinuclear factor
ang	angle
ANG	angiogram, angiography
angio	angiogram
anh	anhydrous
ANLL	acute nonlymphocytic leukemia
annot	annotation
ANoA	anodal opening contraction
ANOVA	analysis of variance
ANP	adult nurse practitioner • advanced nurse practitioner
ANRL	antihypertensive neural renomedullary lipids
ANS	anterior nasal spine • arterionephrosclerosis • autonomic nervous system

ANSI	American National Standards Index • American National Standards Institute
ant	antenna • anterior
ANT	aminonitrothiazol • anterior
antag	antagonist
ante	before *(ante)*
anti-coag	anticoagulant
anti-HAV	antibody to hepatitis A virus
anti-HBc	antibody to hepatitis B core antigen
anti-HBe	antibody to hepatitis Be antigen
anti-HBs	antibody to hepatitis B surface antigen
anti-log	antilogarithm
ant pit	anterior pituitary
ant sup spine	anterior superior spine
ANTU	alpha-naphthylthiourea
ANUG	acute necrotizing ulcerative gingivitis
Ao	aorta
AO	achievement orientation • anodal opening • aortic opening
A+O x 4	alert and oriented to person, place, time and date
AOA	American Osteopathic Association
AOB	alcohol on breath
AOC	abridged ocular chart • anodal opening contraction
AOCl	anodal opening clonus
AOD	arterial occlusive disease
AODM	adult-onset diabetes mellitus
AOL	acro-osteolysis
AOM	acute otitis media
AOMA	American Occupational Medical Association

AONE	American Organization of Nurse Executives
AOO	anodal opening odor
AOP	anodal opening picture
AORN	Association of Operating Room Nurses
aor regurg	aortic regurgitation
aort sten	aortic stenosis
AOS	anodal opening sound
AOTA	American Occupational Therapy Association
AOTe	anodal opening tetanus
AOTF	American Occupational Therapy Foundation
AoV	aortic valve
ap	apothecary • before dinner (*ante prandium*)
AP	acid phosphatase • action potential • alkaline phosphatase • alum-precipitated • angina pectoris • anterior pituitary • anteroposterior • antipyrine • aortic pressure • apical pulse • appendectomy, appendix • arterial pressure • artificial pneumothorax • attending physician • axiopulpal
A/P	ascites-plasma ratio
A&P	anatomy and physiology • anterior and posterior • auscultation and palpation • auscultation and percussion
A$_2$=P$_2$	second aortic sound equals second pulmonic sound
A$_2$>P$_2$	second aortic sound greater than second pulmonic sound
A$_2$<P$_2$	second aortic sound less than second pulmonic sound
APA	Administrative Procedures Act • aldosterone-producing adenoma • American Pharmaceutical Association • American Physiotherapy Association • American Podiatry Association • American Psychiatric Association • antipernicious anemia (factor)
APACHE	acute physiology and chronic health evaluation system

AP/AHC	Accreditation Program/Ambulatory Health Care
APB	atrial premature beat
APC	acute pharyngoconjunctival fever • adenoidal-pharyngeal-conjunctival (virus) • aspirin, phenacetin, caffeine • atrial premature contraction
APC-C	aspirin, phenacetin and caffeine with codeine
APD	action potential duration • anteroposterior diameter
APE	anterior pituitary extract
APF	animal protein factor
APG	ambulatory patient group
A.P.G.A.R.	adaptability, partnership, growth, affection, resolve (family screening - not the same as Apgar scoring systems for newborns)
APH	antepartum hemorrhage • anterior pituitary hormone
APhA	American Pharmaceutical Association
APHA	American Public Health Association
AP/HC	Accreditation Program/Hospice Care
AP/HHC	Accreditation Program/Home Health Care
API	ankle-arm pressure index
APIC	Association for Practitioners in Infection Control
APK	antiparkinsonian
APL	accelerated painless labor • acute promyelocytic leukemia • anterior pituitary-like substance • A Programming Language
AP&L	anteroposterior and lateral
AP&Lat	anteroposterior and lateral
AP/LTC	Accreditation Program/Long Term Care
APN	advanced practice nurse
APO	adverse patient occurrences
APORF	acute postoperative renal failure

app	appendix • applied • approximate
APP	appendix
appar	apparatus • apparent
AP/PF	Accreditation Program/Psychiatric Facilities
appl	appliance • applicable • application • applied
applan	flattened *(applanatus)*
appoint	appointment
approx	approximate
appt	appointment
APPT	Adolescent-Pediatric Pain Tool
appy	appendectomy
APR	abdominoperineal resection • accelerator-produced radiopharmaceuticals • anterior pituitary reaction
aprax	apraxia
APS	acute physiology score • adenosine phosphosulfate • Adult Protective Services
APSAC	anisoylated plasminogen streptokinase activator complex
APT	alum-precipitated toxoid
APTA	American Physical Therapy Association
APTC	ambulatory psoriasis treatment center
APTD	Aid to the Permanently and Totally Disabled
aPTT	activated partial thromboplastin time
APTT	activated partial thromboplastin time
APUD	amine precursor uptake and decarboxylation cells
APVD	anomalous pulmonary venous drainage
aq	aqueous • water *(aqua)*
AQ	accomplishment quotient • achievement quotient • anxiety quotient
aq bull	boiling water *(aqua bulliens)*

aq com	common water *(aqua communis)*
aq dest	distilled water *(aqua destillata)*
aq ferv	hot water *(aqua fervens)*
aq frig	cold water *(aqua frigida)*
aq mar	sea water *(aqua marina)*
aq pur	pure water *(aqua pura)*
aq tep	tepid water *(aqua tepida)*
aqu	aqueous
Ar	argon
AR	abnormal record • achievement ration • active resistance exercises • alarm reaction • analytic reagent • aortic regurgitation • artificial respiration • autosomal recessive
A/R	accounts receivable • apical-radial
Ara	arabinose
ARA	American Rheumatism Association
Ara-A	adenine arabinoside
Ara-C	cytosine arabinoside
ARBOR	arthropod-borne (virus)
ARBOW	artificial rupture of bag of waters
ARC	AIDS-related complex • alcohol rehabilitation center • American Red Cross • American Refugee Committee • anomalous retinal correspondence
Arch	archives
ARD	acute respiratory disease • anorectal dressing • antimicrobial removal device
ARDS	acute respiratory distress syndrome • adult respiratory distress syndrome
ARF	acute renal failure • acute respiratory failure • acute rheumatic fever
ARFC	autorosette-forming cells

arg	silver *(argentum)*
Arg	arginine
ARI	acute respiratory infection
ARM	artificial rupture of membranes
ARMD	age-related macular degeneration
AROM	artificial rupture of membranes
ARP	absolute refractory period
ARRD	Asthma, Rhinitis & other Respiratory Diseases
ARRT	American Registry of Radiologic Technologists
ARS	antirabies serum
ARS-A	arylsulfatase A
art	artery, arterial • artificial
ART	accelerated recovery technique • Accredited Record Technician • automated reagin test
artif	artificial
ARV	AIDS-related virus
As	arsenic
AS	acute salpingitis • androsterone sulfate • ankylosing spondylitis • antiserum • anxiety state • aortic stenosis • aqueous suspension • arteriosclerosis • astigmatism • atrial stenosis • left ear *(auris sinistra)* • sickle cell trait (hemoglobin, genotype)
A-S	Adams-Stokes (disease, syndrome)
A/S	sickle-cell trait (hemoglobin, genotype)
ASA	acetylsalicylic acid (aspirin) • American Society of Anesthesiologists • American Standards Association
ASAP	as soon as possible
ASAS	American Society of Abdominal Surgery • argininosuccinate synthetase
ASC	altered state of consciousness

Asc-A	ascending aorta
ASCH	American Society for Clinical Hypnosis
ASCLT	American Society of Clinical Laboratory Technicians
ASCP	American Society of Clinical Pathologists
ASCVD	arteriosclerotic cardiovascular disease
ASD	aldosterone secretion defect • anterior sagittal diameter • atrial septal defect
ASDC	Association of Sleep Disorders Centers
ASE	axilla, shoulder, elbow
ASET	American Society of Electroencephalographic Technologists
ASF	aniline, sulfur, formaldehyde
AsH	hypermetropic astigmatism
ASH	antistreptococcal hyalurodinase • asymmetric septal hypertrophy
ASHD	arteriosclerotic heart disease
ASHRM	American Society of Hospital Risk Managers
ASIA	American Spinal Injury Association
ASIS	anterior superior iliac spine
ASL	American Sign Language • antistreptolysin
ASLC	acute self-limited colitis
ASL-O	antistreptolysin-O
AsM	myopic astigmatism
ASMI	anteroseptal myocardial infarction
ASMT	American Society for Medical Technology
Asn	asparagine
ASO	antistreptolysin-O
ASOT	antistreptolysin-O titer
Asp	asparagine • aspartate
ASP	area systolic pressure

ASPAN	American Society of Plastic and Reconstructive Surgeons
ASPVD	arteriosclerotic peripheral vascular disease
ASQ	Abbreviated Symptom Questionnaire
ASR	aldosterone secretion rate
ASRT	American Society of Radiologic Technologists
ASS	anterior superior spine
assby	assembly
AS-SCORE	assessing severity: Age of patient, Systems involved, Stage of disease, COmplications, REsponse to therapy
assn	association
assoc	associate, association
asst	assistant
Ast	astigmatism
AST	antistreptolysin titer • Aphasia Screening Test • aspartate aminotransferase
ASTM	American Society for Testing Materials
ASTO	antistreptolysin-O
As tol	as tolerated
ASTR	American Society of Therapeutic Radiologists
ASV	antisiphon valve • anti-snake venom
A-SV	arterial-superficial venous difference
ASVD	arteriosclerotic vascular disease
Asx	asymptomatic
at	airtight • atom
At	astatine
AT	abdominal tympany • achievement test • adjunctive therapy • antithrombin • atraumatic
A-T	ataxia-telangiectasia

AT-III	antithrombin-III
AT$_{10}$	dihydrotachysterol
ATA	alimentary toxic aleukia • atmosphere absolute (pressure at sea level)
ATB	antibiotics • atrial tachycardia with block
ATC	around the clock
ATCC	American Type Culture Collection
ATD	admission, transfer, discharge • antithyroid drugs
at fib	atrial fibrillation
ATG	antithrombocyte globulin
ATH	acute toxic hepatitis
ATL	Achilles tendon lengthening • adult T-cell leukemia • atypical lymphocytes
ATLL	adult T-cell leukemia/lymphoma
ATLS	advanced trauma life support
atm	atmosphere, atmospheric
ATM	acute transverse myelitis
ATN	acute tubular necrosis
AT/NC	atraumatic/normocephalic
at no	atomic number
ATNR	asymmetrical tonic neck reflex
ATP	adenosine triphosphate
ATPase	adenosine triphosphatase
ATPD	ambient temperature and pressure, dry
ATPS	ambient temperature and pressure, saturated
atr	atrophy
ATR	Achilles tendon reflex
ATR FIB	atrial fibrillation
ATS	antitetanic serum • antithymocyte serum • anxiety tension state • atherosclerosis

at wt	atomic weight
Au	gold *(aurum)*
^{198}Au	colloidal gold
AU	Angstrom Unit • antitoxin unit • Australia antigen • both ears *(aures unitas)*, each ear *(auris uterque)*
AUA	American Urological Association
AUC	area under concentration • blood concentration curve (area under the curve)
AUD	auditory
AUL	acute undifferentiated leukemia
aus	auscultation
ausc	auscultation
auscul	auscultation
aux	auxiliary
av	average • avoirdupois
AV	aortic valve • arteriovenous • atrioventricular avoirdupois
AVA	arteriovenous anastomosis
AvCDO$_2$	arteriovenous oxygen content difference
AVD	apparent volume of distribution
avdp	avoirdupois
AVF	augmented voltage unipolar left foot lead (ECG)
AVH	acute viral hepatitis
AVI	air velocity index
AVL	augmented voltage unipolar left arm lead (ECG)
AVM	arteriovenous malformation
AVN	atrioventricular node
A-VO^2	arteriovenous oxygen difference
AVP	antiviral protein

AVR	aortic valve replacement • augmented voltage unipolar right arm lead (ECG)
AVS	arteriovenous shunt
AVT	Allen vision test
AW	anterior wall
A&W	alive and well
AWF	adrenal weight factor
AWHONN	Association for Women's Health, Obstetric and Neonatal Nurses
AWI	anterior wall infarction
AWMI	anterior wall myocardial infarction
AWOL	absent without leave
AWS	alcohol withdrawal syndrome
ax	axilla, axillary • axis, axial
Ax	axilla, axillary
ax grad	axial gradient
Az	nitrogen *(azote)*
AZ	Aschheim-Zondek test
AZT	Aschheim-Zondek test • zidovudine
AzUR	6-azauridine

B

b	twice *(bis)*
B	bacillus • balnium • barometric • base • bath • Baumé scale • behavior • Benoist scale • bicuspid • bilateral • black • blood • blue • body • born • boron • both • brother • buccal • gauss (unit of magnetic induction)
Ba	barium
BA	Bachelor of Arts • bile acid • blood alcohol • boric acid • brachial artery • bronchial asthma • buccoaxial
B/A	backache
BAA	benzoyl arginine amide
BAC	bacterial antigen complex • blood alcohol concentration
BACOP	bleomycin, Adriamycin, cyclophosphamide, oncovin, prednisone
bact	bacteriology • bacterium, bacteria, bacterial
BaEn	barium enema
BAEP	brain-stem auditory evoked potential
BAER	brain-stem auditory evoked response
BAG	buccoaxiogingival
BAIB	beta-aminobutyric acid
bal	balance
BAL	British anti-Lewisite (dimercaprol) • bronchoalveolar lavage
bals	balsam
BaM	barium meal
BAO	basal acid output

BAO/MAO   ratio of basal acid output to maximal acid output

BAP   blood agar plate • brachial artery pressure

bar   barometer, barometric

barbs   barbiturates

BASH   body acceleration synchronous with heartbeat

BASIC   Beginner's All-Purpose Symbolic Instruction Code

baso   basophil

BAT   basic assurance test • best available technology • brown adipose tissue

batt   battery

BB   bath blanket • bed bath • blood bank • both bones • breakthrough bleeding • breast biopsy • buffer base

BBA   Bachelor of Business Administration • born before arrival

BBB   blood-brain barrier • bundle branch block

BBC   brombenzylcyanide

BBS   bilateral breath sounds

BBT   basal body temperature

BC   birth control • blood culture • Blue Cross • board-certified • bone conduction • Bowman's capsule • buccocervical

B&C   board and care

BCAA   branched chain amino acid

BC/BS   Blue Cross/Blue Shield

BCC   basal-cell carcinoma • birth control clinic

BCDDP   Breast Cancer Detection Demonstration Program

BCE   basal-cell epithelioma

BCF   basophil chemotactic factor

BCG   bacillus Calmette-Guérin • ballistocardiogram • bicolor guaiac • bromocresol green

BCH	basal-cell hyperplasia
BCI	Basic and Clinical Immunology
BCLS	basic cardiac life support
BCNU	bischloroethylnitrosourea
BCP	birth control pill • bromocresol purple
BCS	battered child syndrome
bd	twice daily *(bis die)*
BD	base of prism down • basophilic degeneration • bed • benzodiazepine • bile duct • birth defect • board • borderline dull • brain dead • bucco distal
BDC	burn-dressing change
BDE	bile duct exploration
BDS	Bachelor of Dental Surgery
BDSc	Bachelor of Dental Science
Be	Baumé scale • beryllium
BE	*Bacillen Emulsion* • bacterial endocarditis • barium enema • base excess • below elbow • board-eligible
BEAM	Brain Electrical Activity Mapping
BEE	basal energy expenditure
beg	began, begin, beginning
beh	behavior, behavioral
BEI	butanol-extractable iodine
bepti	bionomics, environment, *Plasmodium*, treatment, immunity (malaria epidemiology)
BES	balanced electrolyte solution
bet	between
bev	billion electron-volts
BF	bentonite flocculation • blastogenic factor • blood flow • body fat • bone fragment • boy friend • buffered

B/F	bound-free ratio
BFM	bendroflumethiazide
BFP	biologic false-positive
BFR	blood filtration rate • blood flow rate • bone formation rate
BFR sol	buffered Ringer's solution
BFT	bentonite flocculation test
BFU-E	burst-forming units-erythroid
BG	bicolor guaiac test • blood glucose • Bordet-Gengou (agar, bacillus phenomenon) • buccogingival
BGG	bovine gamma globulin
BH	bill of health • bundle of His
BHA	butylated hydroxyanisole
BHC	benzene hexachloride
BHCDA	Bureau of Health Care Delivery & Assistance
BHI	bone healing index
BHIB	beef heart infusion broth
BHL	biologic half-life
BHP	Bureau of Health Professions
BHRD	Bureau of Health Resources Development
BHS	beta-hemolytic streptococci
BHT	butylated hydroxytoluene
BH/VH	body hematocrit-venous hematocrit ratio
Bi	bismuth
BI	base of prism in • bifocal • bone injury • Braille Institute
bib	drink *(bibe)*
BIB	brought in by
Bicarb	bicarbonate

bid	twice daily *(bis in die)*
BID	brought in dead
blf	bifocal
BIH	benign intracranial hypertension
bihor	during two hours *(bihorium)*
Bi. Isch.	between ischial tuberosities
bil	bilateral • bilirubin
bilat	bilateral
bili	bilirubin
bin	twice a night *(bis in nocte)*
biol	biologic, biology
BIP	background interference procedure • bacterial intravenous protein • biparietal • bismuth iodoform paraffin
BIPP	back injury prevention program • bismuth iodoform paraffin paste
BIR	basic incidence rate
bis	twice *(bis)*
Bi sp	bispinous
bi wk	twice a week
BJ	biceps jerk
B-J	Bence-Jones protein
Bk	berkelium
BK	below knee
BKA	below-knee amputation
BKTT	below knee to toe
BKWC	below knee walking cast
bl	bleeding • blood
BL	blood loss • body lean • buccolingual • Burkitt's lymphoma

BLB	Boothby, Lovelace, Bulbulian (mask)
bl cult	blood culture
bld	blood
BLE	both lower extremities
Bleo	bleomycin
BLESS	bath, laxative, enema, shampoo, shower
BLFG	bilateral firm (hand) grips
BLG	Beta-lactoglobin
BLIP	beta-lactamase inhibitory protein
BLLS	bilateral leg strength
BLM	bleomycin
BLN	bronchial lymph nodes
BlP	blood pressure
BLS	basic life support • blood sugar
BM	Bachelor of Medicine • basal metabolism • basement membrane • bone marrow • bowel movement • buccomesial
BMA	British Medical Association
BMB	bone marrow biopsy
BMC	bone mineral content
BMD	bone marrow depression • Bureau of Medical Devices
BMK	birthmark
BMMP	benign mucous membrane pemphigus
BMN	bone marrow necrosis
BMQA	Board of Medical Quality Assurance
BMR	basal metabolic rate
BMS	Bachelor of Medical Science
BMT	bone marrow transplant
BMZ	basement membrane zone

BNA	*Basle Nomina Anatomica* (nomenclature)
BNDD	Bureau of Narcotics and Dangerous Drugs
BNO	bladder neck obstruction
BO	base of prism out • body odor • bowel • bowels open • bucco-occlusal
B/O	because of
B&O	belladonna and opium
BOA	born out of asepsis
BOB	Bureau of Biologics
BOD	biochemical oxygen demand
BOEA	ethyl biscoumacetate
bol	pill *(bolus)*
BOM	bilateral otitis media
BOR	bowels open regularly
bot	bottle
BOW	bag of waters (amniotic sac)
BP	barometric pressure • bathroom privileges • bedpan • biparietal • birthplace • blood pressure • body part • boiling point • British Pharmacopoeia • bronchopleural • buccopulpal • bypass
BPB	bromphenol blue
BPD	biparietal diameter • blood pressure decreased • bronchopulmonary dysplasia
BPF	bronchopleural fistula
BPH	benign prostatic hypertrophy
BPI	blood pressure increased
BPL	beta-propiolactone
BPM	beats per minute
BPPV	benign paroxysmal positional vertigo
BPRS	Brief Psychiatric Rating Scale

BPV	benign paroxysmal vertigo • benign positional vertigo • bovine papilloma virus
Bq	becquerel
BQA	Board of Quality Assurance • Bureau of Quality Assurance
br	branch • breath • brother
bR	bacteriorhodopsin
Br	bromine • bronchitis • brown
BR	bathroom • bedrest • *Brucella*
BRAT	bananas, rice cereal, applesauce and toast (diet)
BRB	bright red blood
BRBPR	bright red blood per rectum
BRH	Bureau of Radiological Health
BRM	biological response modifier
bronch	bronchoscope, bronchoscopy
BRP	bathroom privileges • bilirubin production
BS	Bachelor of Science • Bachelor of Surgery • barium swallow • blood sugar • bispecific • Blue Shield • bowel sounds • breath sounds
B&S	Bartholin's and Skene's glands
BSA	beef serum albumin • body surface area • bovine serum albumin
BSB	body surface burned • breath sounds bilateral
BSC	bedside commode
BSD	bedside drainage
BSE	breast self-examination
BSER	brain-stem evoked response
BSF	basal skull fracture
BSL	blood sugar level
BSN	Bachelor of Science in Nursing • bowel sounds normal

BSNA	bowel sounds normal and active
BSO	bilateral salpingo-oophorectomy
BSOM	bilateral serous otitis media
BSp	bronchospasm
BSP	bromosulfophthalein
BSPA	bowel sounds present and active
BSPIS	Body Substance Precautions and Isolation Systems
BSR	blood sedimentation rate
BSS	balanced salt solution • black silk suture • buffered saline solution
BST	blood serologic test • brief-stimulus therapy
BSU	British Standard Unit
BSV	Batten-Spielmyer-Vogt(syndrome)
BSW	Bachelor of Social Work
BT	bedtime • bitemporal • bladder tumor • bleeding time • body temperature • brain tumor • bulbotruncal
BTB	breakthrough bleeding • bromthymol blue
BTFS	breast tumor frozen section
BTM	bilateral tympanic membranes
BTPS	body temperature, pressure, saturated
BTS	bioptic telescopic spectacle
BTU	British thermal unit
Bu	bilirubin • butyl
BU	base of prism up • below the umbilicus • Bodansky unit • Burn Unit
bucc	buccal
BUE	both upper extremities
BUN	blood urea nitrogen
BUS	Bartholin's, urethral, and Skene's glands

BV	basilic vein • biological value • blood vessel • blood volume • bulboventricular
B/V	binging and vomiting
B&V	binging and vomiting
BVAD	biventricular assistive device
BVE	biventricular enlargement
BVI	Better Vision Institute
BVRT	Benton Visual Retention Test
BW	below waist • biologic warfare • birth weight • blood Wassermann • body water • body weight
B&W	black and white (cascara and milk of magnesia
BWS	battered woman syndrome
Bx	biopsy
BX	biopsy • Blue Cross
BX/BS	Blue Cross/Blue Shield
Bz-Ty-PABA	benzoyl-tyrosyl-para-aminobenzoic acid (test)

C

c	calorie (small calorie, gram calorie) • capacity • capillary • contact • cubic • curie • cycle • hundred (centum)
$\bar{c}$	with *(cum)*
C	calorie (large calorie, kilocalorie) canine tooth • carbohydrate • carbon • cathode • Caucasian • Celsius • centigrade • cerebrospinal fluid • certified • cervical (nerve, vertebra) • cesarean (section) • chest • cholesterol • clearance • clonus • closure • coarse • cocaine • coefficient • color sense • complement • compound • concentration • content • contraction • cortex • coulomb (electrical unit) • cylinder • cytosine • gallon *(congius)* • hundred *(centum)* • rib *(costa)*
C'	complement
c^2	square centimeter
c^{14}	radioactive carbon
C'-3	component of complement in serum
C1-C7	cervical vertebrae 1 through 7
C1-C9	complements C1 through C9
C-I to C-V	controlled substances-Schedules I thru V
ca	about, approximately *(circa)*
Ca	calcium • cancer • *Candida* • carcinoma • cathode
CA	cancer • carcinoma • cardiac arrest • cholic acid • chronological age • Cocaine Anonymous • cold agglutinin • common antigen • compressed air • conditioned abstinence • coronary artery • cortisone acetate • croup-associated (virus) • cytosine arabinoside

c/a	Clinitest/Acetest
CAAT	computer assisted axial tomography
CAB	coronary artery bypass
CABG	coronary artery bypass graft
CaBP	calcium-binding protein
CAC	cardiac accelerator center • circulating anticoagulant
CaC$_2$	calcium carbide
CaCC	cathodal closure contraction
CaCl$_2$	calcium chloride
CaCO$_3$	calcium carbonate
CaC$_2$O$_4$	calcium oxalate
CACX	cancer of the cervix
CAD	computer-assisted dialogue • coronary artery disease
CaDTe	cathodal duration tetanus
CaEdTA	edathamil calcium disodium
CAF	contract administration fees • cyclophosphamide, Adriamycin, fluorouracil
CAG	chronic atrophic gastritis
CAH	chronic active hepatitis • chronic aggressive hepatitis • congenital adrenal hyperplasia
CAI	computer-assisted instruction • confused artificial insemination
cal	caliber • calorie (small or gram calorie)
Cal	calorie (large calorie, kilocalorie)
C$_{alb}$	albumin clearance
calc	calculate, calculated
CALD	chronic active liver disease
calef	warmed (*calefactus*)
CALLA	common acute lymphocytic leukemia antigen
C$_{am}$	amylase clearance

CAM	chorioallantoic membrane
cAMP	cyclic adenosine monophosphate
c amplum	heaping spoonful, tablespoonful *(cochleare amplum)*
CAN	*Candida* • cord (umbilical) around neck
canc	canceled
CaO	calcium oxide (quick lime)
CAO	chronic airway obstruction
CaO$_2$	arterial oxygen content
CaOC	cathodal opening contraction
Ca(OH)$_2$	calcium hydroxide
ca ox	calcium oxalate
cap	capacity • capillary • capsule • community action program • let him take *(capiat)*
CAP	choramphenicol • College of American Pathologists • Computerized Automated Psychophysiological (device)
CAPD	continuous ambulatory peritoneal dialysis
cardiol	cardiology
CAS	cerebral arteriosclerosis • Chemistry Abstract Service • chronic anovulation syndrome
CaSO$_4$	calcium sulfate
CASS	Coronary Artery Surgery Study
CAT	cataract • Children's Apperception Test • chronic abdominal tympany • computerized axial tomography
cath	cathartic • catheter, catheterize, catheterization • cathode
cauc	Caucasian
cav	cavity
CAV	congenital absence of vagina • congenital adrenal virilism • croup-associated virus
Cb	columbium

CB	Bachelor of Surgery *(Chirurgiae Baccalaureus)* ceased breathing • chronic bronchitis
C-B	chest-back
CBA	chronic bronchitis with asthma
CBBB	complete bundle branch block
CBC	complete blood count
CBCME	computer-based continuing medical education
CBD	closed bladder drainage • common bile duct
CBF	capillary blood flow • cerebral blood flow
CBG	corticosteroid-binding globulin • cortisol-binding globulin
CBO	Congressional Budget Office
CBOC	completion of bed occupancy care
CBR	carotid bodies resected • chemical, bacteriologic and radiologic • complete bed rest • crude birth rate
CBS	chronic brain syndrome
CBV	circulating blood volume
CBW	chemical and biological warfare
CBZ	carbamazepine
CBZE	carbamazepine epoxide
cc	cubic centimeter
CC	cell culture • cellular compartment • chief (current) complaint • circulatory collapse • coefficient of correlation certified • complications and co-morbidities • compound cathartic • concave • cord compression • coronary collateral • corpus callosum • costochondral • critical condition • current complaint
C&C	confirmed and compatible
CCA	chick-cell agglutination • chimpanzee coryza agent • cholangiocarcinoma • circumflex coronary artery • common carotid artery • congenital contractual arachnodactyly

CCAT	conglutinating complement absorption test
CCB	calcium channel blockers
CCBV	central circulating blood volume
CCC	cathodal closure contraction • central counteradaptive changes • chronic calculous cholecystitis
CCCR	closed chest cardiac resuscitation
CCD	calibration curve data • charge-coupled device
CCF	cephalin-cholesterol flocculation (test) • congestive cardiac failure
CCI	chronic coronary insufficiency
CCK	cholecystokinin
CCK-GB	cholecystokinin-gallbladder (cholecystogram)
CCK-PZ	cholecystokinin-pancreozymin
CCME	Coordinating Council for Medical Education
CCMS	clean-catch midstream
CCMSUA	clean-catch midstream urinalysis
CCNS	cell-cycle nonspecific (agent)
CCNSC	Cancer Chemotherapy National Service Center
CCNU	chloroethylcyclohexylnitrosourea (lomustine)
CCP	Crippled Children's Program
CCPD	continuous cycled peritoneal dialysis
C$_{cr}$	creatine clearance
CCRC	continuing care retirement community
CCRN	Certified Critical Care Registered Nurse
CCS	casualty clearing station • cell-cycle specific (agent) • Critical Care Services
cct	circuit
CCT	carotid compression tomography • chocolate-coated tablet • closed cerebral trauma • coated compressed tablet • controlled cord traction

CCTe	cathodal closure tetanus
CCU	cardiac care unit • coronary care unit
CCW	counterclockwise
cd	caudal
Cd	cadmium • coccygeal
CD	cardiovascular deconditioning • cardiovascular disease • caudal • cesarean-delivered • cesarean delivery • chemical dependency • civil defense • common duct • communicable disease • constant drainage • contagious disease • convulsive disorder • Crohn's disease • curative dose • current diagnosis • cystic duct • diagonal conjugate diameter of pelvic inlet *(conjugata diagonalis)*
C&D	cystoscopy and dilatation
CD$_{50}$	median curative dose
CDA	congenital dyserythropoietic anemia
CDAA	chlorodiallylacetamide
C&DB	cough and deep breathe
CDC	calculated day of confinement • Centers for Disease Control
CDCA	chenodeoxycholic acid
CDE	canine distemper encephalitis • Certified Diabetes Educator • common duct exploration
CDH	congenital dislocation of hip
CDNA	complementary deoxyribonucleic acid • copy deoxyribonucleic acid
CDP	comprehensive discharge planning • constant distending pressure • cytidine diphosphate • cytidine diphosphocholine
CDS	cul-de-sac
CDT	carbon dioxide therapy
Cdyn	dynamic compliance
Ce	cerium

CE	California encephalitis • cardiac enlargement • cardiac enzyme • cerebral embolus • chloroform-ether • cholesterol esters • clinical emphysema • conjugated estrogens • constant error • continuing education • stroke
CEA	carcinoembryonic antigen • crystalline egg albumin
CED	chronic enthusiasm disorder • chronic erythema disorder • cultural/ethnic diversity
CEEV	Central European encephalitis virus
CEF	chick embryo fibroblast (vaccine)
Cel	Celsius
CELO	chick embryo lethal orphan (virus)
CEM	conventional-transmission electron microscope
cemf	counter-electromotive force
CEN	Certified Emergency Nurse
cent	centigrade • central
CEO	chick embryo origin • chief executive officer
CEP	congenital erythropoietic porphyria • counter-electrophoresis • counterimmunoelectrophoresis
Ceph-floc	cephalin flocculation (test)
CEQ	Council on Environmental Quality
CER	capital expenditure review • conditioned emotional response
cert	certificate • certified
cerv	cervical
CES	central excitatory state
CEU	continuing education unit
cf	compare *(confer)*
Cf	californium • iron *(ferrum)* • carrier

CF	carbolfuchsin • cardiac failure • chest and left leg • Christmas factor • citrovorum factor complement fixation • contractile force • count fingers (visual acuity test) • cystic fibrosis
C'F	complement fixing
C/F	count fingers (visual acuity test)
CFA	complement-fixing antibody • complete Freund adjuvant
CFC	colony-forming cell • continuous-flow centrifugation
CFF	critical fusion frequency (test) • Cystic Fibrosis Foundation
CFFA	cystic fibrosis factor activity
Cf-Fe	carrier-bound iron (*ferrum*)
CFI	chemotactic factor inactivator • complement fixation inhibition test
CFO	chief financial officer
CFR	Code of Federal Regulations
CFS	cancer family syndrome
CFT	complement fixation test
CFU	colony-forming unit
CFU-C	colony-forming unit-culture
CFU-E	colony-forming unit-erythroid
CFU-S	colony-forming unit-spleen
CFW	cancer-free white (mouse)
cg	centigram
CG	center of gravity • cholecystogram, cholecystography • chorionic gonadotropin • chronic glomerulonephritis • colloidal gold • control group • phosgene ("choking gas")
CGC	Certified Gastrointestinal Clinician
CGD	chromosomal gonadal dysgenesis • chronic granulomatous disease

CGH	chorionic gonadotropic hormone
CGL	chronic granulocytic anemia • chronic granulocytic leukemia
cgm	centigram
CGM	central gray matter
cGMP	cyclic guanosine monophosphate
CGN	chronic glomerulonephritis • Convalescent Growing Nursery
CGP	chorionic growth-hormone prolactin
cgs	centimeter-gram-second (system)
CGS	catgut suture • centimeter-gram-second (system)
CGTT	cortisone-glucose tolerance test
ch	chest • chief • child • chronic
CH	cholesterol • convalescent hospital • crown-heel length
C&H	cocaine and heroin
CHA	congenital hypoplastic anemia
ChAc	choline acetyltransferase
CHAMPUS	Civilian Health and Medical Program of the Uniformed Services
CHAMPVA	Civilian Health and Medical Program of the Veterans Administration
CHAP	Child Health Assessment Program
chart	a paper *(charta)*
ChB	Bachelor of Surgery *(Chirurgiae Baccalaureus)*
CHB	complete heart block
CHC	Community Health Center
ChD	Doctor of Surgery *(Chirurgiae Baccalaureus)*
ChE	cholinesterase
chem	chemical, chemistry
CHEOPS	Children's Hospital of Eastern Ontario Pain Scale

CHF	congestive heart failure
chg	change
CHI	creatinine height index
CHIP	Comprehensive Health Insurance Plan
chl	chloroform
CHL	chloramphenicol
ChM	Master of Surgery (*Chirurgiae Magister*)
CHN	Certified Hemodialysis Nurse • community health network • community health nurse
CHO	carbohydrate
CH₂O	carbohydrate
Chol	cholesterol
CHP	child psychiatry • comprehensive health plan
ch px	chicken pox
chr	chronic
chron	chronic
CHS	Chediak-Higashi syndrome
CHSS	Cooperative Health Statistics System
Ci	curie
CI	cardiac index • cardiac insufficiency • cerebral infarction • chain-initiating chemotherapeutic index • coefficient of intelligence • colloidal iron • Colour Index • crystalline insulin
cib	food (*cibus*)
CIBD	chronic inflammatory bowel disease
CIB HA	congenital inclusion-body hemolytic anemia
CIC	cardiac inhibitor center • Certified Infection Control • circulating immune complex (titer)
CICU	cardiac (coronary) intensive care unit
CID	Central Institute for the Deaf • chick infective dose • cytomegalic inclusion disease

CIDS	cellular immunodeficiency syndrome
CIE	counterimmunoelectrophoresis
CIEP	counterimmunoelectrophoresis
CIF	claims inquiry form • cloning inhibiting factor
CIH	carbohydrate-induced hyperglycemia
CIL	Center for Independent Living • Central Identification Laboratory
CILHI	Central Identification Laboratory - Hawaii
CIM	cortically induced movement
C$_{in}$	insulin clearance
C In	insulin clearance
CIN	cerebriform intradermal nevus • cervical intraepithelial neoplasia • Computers in Nursing
circ	circular • circumcision • circumference
Circ	circulating, circulation, circulatory
CIRR	cirrhosis
CIS	carcinoma in situ • central inhibitory state • clinical information systems
cit	citrate
CIT	combined intermittent therapy
CIV	continuous intravenous (infusion)
CJD	Creutzfeldt-Jakob disease
ck	check
CK	creatine kinase
CK-BB	isoenzyme of creatine kinase with brain subunits
CK-MB	isoenzyme of creatine kinase with muscle and brain subunits
CK-MM	isoenzyme of creatine kinase with muscle subunits
cl	centiliter • clavicle • clinic • closure • corpus luteum
Cl	chloride • chlorine

CL	capacity of the lung • chest and left arm • *Clostridium* • corpus luteum • critical list • current liabilities • cycle length
C$_L$	compliance of the lungs
CLA	cervicolinguoaxial
CLAS	career ladder advancement system
CLBBB	complete left bundle branch block
CL/CP	cleft lip, cleft palate
CLD	chronic liver disease
CLH	chronic lobular hepatitis
clin	clinic, clinical
CLIP	cerebral lipidosis without visceral involvement and with onset of disease past infancy • corticotrophin-like intermediate lobe peptide
CLL	cholesterol-lowering lipid • chronic lymphatic leukemia • chronic lymphocytic leukemia
CLMA	Clinical Laboratory Management Association
CLML	Current List of Medical Literature
CLN	computer liaison nurse
CLO	cod liver oil
CIP	Clinical Pathology
Cl pal	cleft palate
CLS	clinical laboratory scientist
CLSP	clinical laboratory specialist
CLT	clinical laboratory technician • clinical laboratory technologist • clot lysis time
clysis	hypodermoclysis
cm	centimeter • complications • costal margin • tomorrow morning *(cras mane)*
Cm	curium
C$_m$	maximum clearance

CM	case manager • chloroquine and mepacrine • chondromalacia • circular muscle • competing message • congenital malformation • contrast media • costal margin • Master of Surgery
C&M	cocaine and morphine
cm^3	cubic centimeter
CMA	Canadian Medical Association • certified medical assistant
c magnum	tablespoon, tablespoonful *(cochleare magnum)*
CMB	carbolic methylene blue
CMC	carboxymethylcellulose • carpometacarpal • Chloromycetin
CME	cervical mediastinal exploration • continuing medical education • cystoid macular edema
CMF	cyclophosphamide, methotrexate, fluorouracil
CMFP	cyclophosphamide, methotrexate, fluorouracil, prednisone
CMFVP	cyclophosphamide, methotrexate, fluorouracil, vincristine, prednisone
CMG	cystometrogram
CMGN	chronic membranous glomerulonephritis
CMHC	Community Mental Health Center
CMI	carbohydrate metabolism index • cell-mediated immunity • Cornell Medical Index
CMID	cytomegalic inclusion disease
c/min	cycles per minute
CMIR	cell-mediated immune response
CMIT	Current Medical Information and Terminology
CML	cell-mediated lympholysis • chronic myelocytic leukemia • chronic myelogenous leukemia
cmm	cubic millimeter
cm/m^2	centimeters per square meter

CMM	cutaneous malignant melanoma
CMN	cystic medial necrosis
cMo	centimorgan
CMO	cardiac minute output
C-MOPP	cyclophosphamide, mechlorethamine, Oncovin, procarbazine, prednisone
CMP	competitive medical plans • cytidine monophosphate
CMR	cerebral metabolic rate • cystic medial necrosis
CMRG	cerebral metabolic rate of glucose
CMRNG	chromosomally mediated resistant *Neisseria gonorrhoeae*
CMRO	cerebral metabolic rate of oxygen
cms	to be taken tomorrow morning *(cras mane sumendus)*
CMSC	Certified Medical Staff Coordinator
cm/sec	centimeters per second
CMSS	Council of Medical Specialty Societies
CMSUA	clean, midstream urinalysis
CMT	catechol-O-methyltransferase • Charcot-Marie-Tooth • Current Medical Terminology
CMV	cytomegalovirus
cn	tomorrow night *(cras nocte)*
CN	caudate nucleus • Charge Nurse • clinical nursing • congenital nystagmus • cranial nerve • cyanogen
CNA	Canadian Nurses Association • certified nurse assistant • chart not available
CNE	chronic nervous exhaustion
CNH	community nursing home
CNL	community nursing liaison
CNM	certified nurse-midwife • clinical nurse manager

CNOR	Certified Nurse, Operating Room
CNP	constant negative pressure
CNRN	Certified Neuroscience Registered Nurse
cns	to be taken tomorrow night *(cras nocte sumendus)*
CNS	central nervous system • clinical nurse-specialist • computerized notation system
CNSD	chronic nonspecific diarrhea
CNSN	Certified Nutrition Support Nurse
CNV	contingent negative variation
co	cutoff
Co	cobalt • coenzyme
^{60}Co	radioactive cobalt
CO	carbon monoxide • cardiac output • castor oil • co-insurance • compound • cross-over
C/O	complains of
CO_2	carbon dioxide
Co I	coenzyme I (diphosphopyridine nucleotide, nicotinamide adenine dinucleotide)
Co II	coenzyme II (triphosphopyridine nucleotide, nicotinamide adenine dinucleotide phosphate)
CoA	coenzyme A
COAD	chronic obstructive airway disease
coag	coagulation
COAP	cyclophosphamide, Oncovin, cytosine arabinoside, prednisone
COB	coordination of benefits
COBOL	Common Business Oriented Language
COBRA	Consolidated Omnibus Budget Reconciliation Act (1985)
COBS	Cesarean-obtained barrier-sustained
COBT	chronic obstruction of biliary tract

coc	coccygeal • coccyx
COC	cathodal opening contraction • combination of oral contraceptive
cochl	spoonful *(cochleare)*
cochl amp	heaping spoonful *(cochleare amplum)*
cochl mag	tablespoonful *(cochleare magnum)*
cochl parv	teaspoonful *(cochleare parvum)*
COCL	cathodal opening clonus
coct	boiling *(coctio)*
cod	codeine
COD	cause of death • chemical oxygen demand • condition on discharge
CODA	Cadaveric Organ Donor Act • Co-Dependents Anonymous
coef	coefficient
coeff	coefficient
COEPS	cortically originating extrapyramidal system
C of A	coarctation of aorta
COGTT	cortisone-primed oral glucose tolerance test
COH	carbohydrate
COHb	carboxyhemoglobin
COHgb	carboxyhemoglobin
col	colony • color • strain (cola)
COL	cost of living
colat	strained *(colatus)*
COLD	chronic obstructive lung disease
cold agg	cold agglutinin
coll	collect, collection • college • colloidal • eyewash *(collyrium)*
collut	mouthwash *(collutorium)*

collyr	eyewash *(collyrium)*
COM	cyclophosphamide, Oncovin, methotrexate
COMA	cyclophosphamide, Oncovin, methotrexate, cytosine arabinoside
comb	combination
ComC	Committee Chairperson
COMLA	cyclophosphamide, Oncovin, methotrexate, leucovorin, cytosine arabinoside
comm	committee, commission, commissioner
commun dis	communicable disease
comp	compare, comparative, comparable • composition • compound • compression
compd	compound
compet	competition
compl	complete, completed • complication
complic	complicating, complication
COMT	catechol-O-methyltransferase
CON	certificate of need
conc	concentrated, concentration
concis	cut *(concisus)*
cond	condense, condensed • condition
cond ref	conditioned reflex
cond resp	conditioned response
conf	conference
cong	congenital • congress • gallon *(conglius)*
congen	congenital
congr	congruent
conjug	conjugated, conjugation
cons	keep *(conserva)*

const	constant
cont	containing • contents • continue, continued
cont rem	let the medicine be continued *(continuatur remedium)*
contrx	contraction
conv ·	convalescent, convalescence
coord	coordination
COP	capillary osmotic pressure • colloid osmotic pressure
COPD	chronic obstructive pulmonary disease
COPE	chronic obstructive pulmonary emphysema
COPP	cyclophosphamide, Oncovin, procarbazine, prednisone
coq	boil *(coque)*
CoQ	coenzyme Q
coq in s a	boil in sufficient water *(coque in sufficiente aqua)*
coq s a	boil properly *(coque secundum artem)*
cor	corrected • heart *(cor)*
CoR	Congo red
COR	Comprehensive Outpatient Rehabilitation Facility • coronary • heart *(cor)*
corr	correct, corrected • correlate
cort	Cortex, cortical
CORT	Certified Operating Room Technician
cos	change of shift • cosine
CO$_2$T	total carbon dioxide content
COTA	Certified Occupational Therapy Assistant
COTe	cathodal opening tetanus
COTH	Council of Teaching Hospitals
COTRANS	Coordinated Transfer Application System
coul	coulomb (electrical unit)

cp	chemically pure
CP	candle power • capillary pressure • cerebellopontile • cerebellopontine • cerebral palsy • chemically pure • chloropurine • chloroquine and primaquine • chronic pyelonephritis • cleft palate • clinical pathways • constant pressure • coproporphyrin • cor pulmonale • creatine phosphate • critical pathways • cyclophosphamide
C&P	cystoscopy and pyelogram
CPA	Canadian Physiotherapy Association • cardiopulmonary arrest • carotid phonoangiography, costophrenic angle
CPAN	Certified Post-Anesthesia Nurse
C$_{pah}$	Para-aminohippurate clearance
CPA/OBG	carotid phonoangiography/oculoplethysmography
CPAP	continuous (constant) positive airway pressure
c parvum	teaspoonful (cochleare parvum)
CPB	cardiopulmonary bypass • competitive protein binding
CPBA	competitive protein-binding analysis • competitive protein-binding assay
CPBS	cardiopulmonary bypass surgery
CPC	chronic passive congestion • clinical pathologic correlation • clinicopathologic conference • community psychiatric center
cpd	compare • compound
CPD	cephalopelvic disproportion • citrate phosphate dextrose solution
CPD-A	citrate phosphate dextrose-adenine solution
CPDD	calcium pyrophosphate deposition disease
CPE	chronic pulmonary emphysema • cytopathic effect • cytopathogenic effect
CPEHS	Consumer Protection and Environmental Health Service

CPF	clot-promoting factor
CPGN	chronic progressive glomerulonephritis
CPH	Certificate in Public Health • chronic persistent hepatitis
CPHA	Committee on Professional and Hospital Activities • community public health agency
CPHQ	Certified Professional in Healthcare Quality
CPI	constitutional psychopathic inferiority • consumer price index • coronary prognostic index • cost-patient index
CPIB	chlorophenoxyisobutyrate
CPID	chronic pelvic inflammatory disease
CPK	creatine phosphokinase
CPK-BB (CPK$_1$)	a CPK isoenzyme (CPK$_1$)
CPK-MB (CPK$_2$)	a CPK isoenzyme (CPK$_2$)
CPK-MM (CPK$_3$)	a CPK isoenzyme (CPK$_3$)
cpm	counts per minute
CPM	continuous passive motion • counts per minute
CPMG	Carr-Purcell-Meiboom-Gill (spin-echo technique)
CPN	chronic polyneuropathy • chronic pyelonephritis
CPNP	Certified Pediatric Nurse Practitioner
CPP	cerebral perfusion pressure • cyclopentenopehnanthrene
CPPB	continuous (constant) positive-pressure breathing
CPPD	calcium pyrophosphate dihydrate
CP&PD	chest percussion and postural drainage
CPPV	continuous (constant) positive-pressure ventilation
CPQA	Certified Professional in Quality Assurance

CPR	cardiac and pulmonary rehabilitation • cardiopulmonary resuscitation • computer-based patient records • cortisol production rate
cps	counts per second • cycles per second
CPS	Child Protective Services • chloroquine, pyrimethamine, sulfisoxazole
CPSC	Consumer Product Safety Commission
CPT	chest physiotherapy • combining power test • Current Procedural Terminology
CPT-4	Current Procedural Terminology
CPU	central processing unit (computer)
CPX	complete physical examination
CPZ	chlorpromazine • Compazine
CQ	chloroquine and quinine
CQI	continuous quality improvement
Cr	chromium • creatinine • crisis
CR	cardiorespiratory • central ray • chest and right arm • closed reduction • clot retraction • coefficient of fat retention • colon resection • complete remission • complete response • conditioned reflex, response • controlled-release • cranial creatinine • cresol red • critical ratio • crown-rump (length) • cyanosis retinae
CRA	central retinal artery
CRAB	Central Registry at Bethesda
CRBBB	complete right bundle branch block
CRC	colorectal carcinoma
CRD	chronic renal disease • chronic respiratory disease • completely randomized design • complete reaction of degeneration
CRE	cumulative radiation effect
creat	creatinine

CREST	calcinosis cutis, Raynaud's phenomenon, esophageal dysfunction hypermotility, sclerodactyly, telangiectasia (syndrome)
CRF	chronic renal failure • citrovorum rescue factor • corticotropin-releasing factor
CRH	corticotropin-releasing hormone
crit	criteria • critical
Crit	hematocrit
CRL	crown-rump length
CRM	certified raw milk • cross-reacting material
CRNA	Certified Registered Nurse - Anesthetist
CRO	cathode-ray oscilloscope
CROS	contralateral routing of signal
CrP	creatine phosphate
CRP	community resource professional • C-reactive protein • cystic retinal pigmentation
CRPA	C-reactive protein antiserum
CRS	Chinese restaurant syndrome • colon-rectal surgery • congenital rubella syndrome
CRST	calcinosis cutis, Raynaud's phenomenon, sclerodactyly, telangiectasia (syndrome)
CRT	cathode-ray tube • certified • complex reaction time • community resource trainee
CRTT	certified respiratory therapy technician
CRV	central retinal vein
CRVO	central retinal vein occlusion
crys	crystal, crystalline, crystallized
cryst	crystal, crystalline, crystallized
cs	case • conscious • consciousness
Cs	cesium
^{137}Cs	radioactive cesium

CS	cat scratch • central supply • cesarean section • chronic schizophrenia • clinical stage • completed stroke • conditioned stimulus • conjunctival secretions • coronary sinus • corpus striatum • corticosteroid • current strength • cycloserine
C&S	conjunctiva and sclera • culture and sensitivity • culture and susceptibility
CSB	chemical stimulation of the brain
CSBO	complete small bowel obstruction
CSCT	comprehensive support care team
CSD	cat scratch disease • celiac sprue disease
C-section	Cesarean section
CSF	cerebrospinal fluid • colony-stimulating factor
CSFP	cerebrospinal fluid pressure
CSF-WR	cerebrospinal fluid - Wassermann reaction
CSI	cholesterol saturation index
CSLU	chronic stasis leg ulcer
CSM	cerebrospinal meningitis • circulation, sensation, mobility • Consolidated Standards Manual
CSN	carotid sinus nerve • Certified School Nurse
CSNR	carotid sinus nerve resection
CSNS	carotid sinus nerve stimulation • carotid sinus nerve stimulator
CSOM	chronic serous otitis media
C-spine	cervical spine
CSR	central supply room • Cheyne-Stokes respiration • corrected sedimentation rate • cortisol secretion rate
CSS	chewing, sucking, swallowing
Cst	static compliance
CST	contraction stress test • convulsive shock therapy

CSU	catheter specimen of urine
CSUF	continuous slow ultrafiltration
CT	calcitonin • cardiothoracic • cerebral thrombosis • chemotherapy • circulation time • clotting time • coated tablet • compressed tablet • computerized tomography • connective tissue • Coombs' test • corneal transplant • coronary thrombosis • corrective therapy • crutch training • cytotechnologist
CTA	clear to auscultation • clinical teaching associate • cytoplasmic tubular aggregates • cytotoxic assay
CTAB	cetyltrimethylammonium bromide
CTB	ceased to breathe • chronic tuberculosis
CTBM	cetyltrimethylammonium bromide
CTC	chlortetracycline
CTCL	cutaneous T-cell lymphoma
CTD	carpal tunnel decompression
CTF	Colorado tick fever
C/TG	cholesterol - triglyceride ratio
CTICU	cardiothoracic intensive care unit
CTP	cytidine triphosphate
ctr	center • control
CTR	cardiothoracic ratio
CTS	carpal tunnel syndrome • composite treatment score • computerized tomographic scanner
CTU	cardiothoracic unit • centigrade thermal unit
CTUWSD	chest tube under water seal drainage
CTX	Cytoxan • cervical traction
CTZ	chemoreceptor trigger zone • chlorothiazide
cu	cubic, curie
CU$_\mu$	cubic micron
Cu	copper *(cuprum)*

C_u	urea clearance
CU	cause unknown • clinical unit • control unit • convalescent unit • curie
CUC	chronic ulcerative colitis
cu cm	cubic centimeter
CUD	congenital urinary (tract) deformities
cu ft	cubic foot
CUG	cystourethrogram
cu in	cubic inch
cuj	of which *(cujus)*
cuj lib	of any you desire *(cujus libet)*
cult	culture
cu m	cubic meter
cum	cumulative report
cu mm	cubic millimeter
cur	curative • current
CUR	cystourethrocele
CURN	Certified Urological Registered Nurse
cu yd	cubic yard
cv	tomorrow evening *(cras vespere)*
CV	cardiovascular • cell volume • central venous • cerebrovascular • closing volume • coefficient of variation • concentrated volume • conduction velocity • conjugate diameter of pelvic inlet • constant volume • corpuscular volume • cresyl violet • critical value • curriculum vitae
CVA	cardiovascular accident • cerebrovascular accident • costovertebral angle
CVC	central venous catheter • crying vital capacity
CVD	cardiovascular disease • cerebrovascular disease • color-vision deviant
CVI	cerebrovascular insufficiency

CVN	central venous nutrient
CVO	obstetric conjugate diameter of pelvic inlet (*conjugata vera obstetrica*)
CvO₂	mixed venous oxygen content
CVP	cardiac valve procedure • central venous pressure • cyclophosphamide, vincristine, prednisone
CVP lab	cardiovascular-pulmonary laboratory
CVPP	cyclophosphamide, vincristine, prednisone, procarbazine
CVPR	central venous pressure report
CVR	cardiovascular-renal • cardiovascular-respiratory • cerebrovascular resistance
CVS	cardiovascular surgery • cardiovascular system • chorionic villi sampling • clean-voided specimen
cw	cell wall • common wart • continuous-wave
CW	Case Worker • chemical warfare • chest wall • Children's Ward • clockwise • continuous-wave • crutch walking
CWBTS	capillary whole-blood true sugar
cwop	childbirth without pain
CWP	childbirth without pain • coal workers' pneumoconiosis
CWS	cold water soluble
cwt	hundredweight
Cx	cervix • convex
CXR	chest x-ray
CY	calendar year • cyanogen
c/y	Children and Youth Project of Maternal and Child Health Program
CYCLO	cyclophosphamide • cyclopropane
Cyd	cytidine
cyl	cylinder, cylindrical

CYL	casein yeast lactate
Cys	cysteine • cystoscopy
cysto	cystoscopy
Cyt	Cytosine
cytol	cytologic, cytology
CZI	crystalline zinc insulin

D

d	date • day • deceased, dead, died • degree • density • deuterium • dextro- (right, clockwise) • dose • give (da)
/d	daily, per day
D	date • daughter • day • dead space • deciduous • decreased • density • dermatologist, dermatology • deuterium • deviation • dextrorotatory • dextrose • diameter • died • diffusion coefficient • diopter • disease • distal • diverticulum • divorced • dorsal • dorsal vertebra • dose • duration • right *(dexter)* • vitamin D unit
DA	degenerative arthritis • delayed action • developmental age • direct admission • direct agglutination • disability assistance • dispense as directed • dopamine • ductus arteriosus
D/A	date of admission
DAB	diaminobutyric acid • dimethylaminoazobenzene
DADDS	diacetyldiaminodiphenyl sulfone
DAFT	Draw-a-Family Test
DAGT	direct antiglobulin test
DAH	disordered action of the heart
dal	decaliter
DALA	delta-aminolevulinic acid
DAM	degraded amyloid • diacetylmonoxime
dAMP	deoxyadenosine monophosphate (deoxyadenylate)
DAO	diamine oxidase
DAP	Department of Applied Physiology • dihydroxyacetone phosphate • Draw-a-Person Test

DAPT	direct agglutination pregnancy test • Draw-a-Person Test
DAR	daily affective rhythm
DARP	drug abuse rehabilitation program
DASP	double antibody solid phase
DAT	delayed action tablet • diet as tolerated • differential agglutination titer • differential aptitude test • diphtheria antitoxin • direct antiglobulin test
dau	daughter
DAUNO	daunorubicin
db	decibel
dB	decibel
DB	date of birth • dextran blue • distobuccal
D/B	date of birth
DBA	dibenzanthracene
DBCL	dilute blood clot lysis (method)
DBE	synthetic estrogen
DBF	disturbed bowel function
DBH	dopamine beta-hydroxylase
DBI	development at birth index • phenformin
DBI-TD	phenformin hydrochloride
dbl	double
DBM	diabetic management
DBMS	data-base management system
DBO	distobucco-occlusal
DBP	diastolic blood pressure • dibutylphthalate • distobuccopulpal
dc	discontinue

DC	Dental Corps • diagnostic center • diagonal conjugate • dihydrocodeine • dephenylarsine cyanide • direct Coombs' (test) • direct current • Direction Circular • discharge(d) • discontinue • distocervical • Doctor of Chiropractic • donor cells
D/C	diarrhea/constipation • discontinue
D&C	dilatation and curettage
DCA	deoxycholate-citrate agar • desoxycorticosterone acetate
DCB	dilutional cardiopulmonary bypass
DC&B	dilation, curettage, and biopsy
DCc	double concave
DCC	day care center
DCCN	Dimensions of Critical-Care Nursing
DCCT	Diabetes Control and Complications Trial
DCF	day care facility • direct centrifugal flotation method
DCG	desoxycorticosterone glucoside • disodium cromoglycate
DCH	delayed cutaneous hypersensitivity
DCI	dichloroisoproterenol
DCN	delayed conditioned necrolysis
DCP	dicalcium phosphate • discharge plan, discharge planner
DCR	direct cortical response • direct critical response
DCT	direct Coombs' test • distal convoluted tubule
DCTMA	desoxycorticosterone trimethylacetate
DCTPA	desoxycorticosterone triphenylacetate
DCU	Diabetes Care Unit
DCx	double coverage

DD	dependent drainage • developmental disability • diaper dermatitis • disability determination • disc diameter • differential diagnosis • DiGuglielmo disease • double dose • dry dressing
DDA	DDT metabolite excreted in urine
DDAVP	desamino-D-arginine vasopressin
DDB	donor directed blood
DDC	diethyldithiocarbamic acid
DDD	degenerative disc disease • dense-deposit disease • dichloro-diphenyl-dichloroethane
DDE	DDT metabolite that accumulates in fatty tissue • direct data entry
DDGB	double-dose gallbladder (cholecystogram)
DDR	discharged during referral
DDS	diaminodiphenylsulfone • Doctor of Dental Surgery • dystrophy-dystonia syndrome
DDSc	Doctor of Dental Science
DDST	Denver Developmental Screening Test
DDT	dichloro-diphenyl-trichloroethane (chlorophenothane)
DDVP	dichlorovinyl-dimethyl-phosphate (dichlorvos)
DDx	differential diagnosis
DE	digestive energy • dose equivalent
D&E	dilatation and evacuation
DEA	dehydroepiandrosterone • Drug Enforcement Administration
DEAE	diethylaminothanol • diethylaminoethyl
DEAE-D	diethylaminoethyl dextran
DEB	diethylbutanediol • dystrophic epidermolysis bullosa
DEBA	diethylbarbituric acid
debil	debility
dec	deceased • decompose, decomposed • decreased • pour off (*decanta*)

deca-	ten
dec'd	deceased
decel	deceleration
deci-	one-tenth
decoct	decoction
decomp	decompose, decomposed, decomposition
decr	decrease, decreased
decub	lying down (*decubitus*)
de d in d	from day to day (*de die in diem*)
def	defecate, defecation • deficient, deficiency • definite • definition
DEF	decayed, extracted or filled (teeth)
defic	deficiency
defib	defibrillate
deform	deformity
deg	degeneration • degree
degen	degeneration
deglut	let it be swallowed (*deglutiatur*)
DEHS	Division of Emergency Health Services
del	delivery • delusion
Dem	Demerol (meperidine)
DEM	Department of Emergency Medicine
denom	denominator
dent	dental • let it be given (*dentur*)
dep	dependent
DEP	diethylpropanediol
depr	depressed, depression
dept	department
De R	reaction of degeneration

deriv	derive, derivation, derivative
derm	dermatology, dermatologist
DEM	diethylstilbesterol
desat	desaturation
desc	descent, descending
DESI	Drug Efficacy Study Implementation
dest	distilled *(destillata)*
det	determine • let it be given *(detur)*
DET	diethyltryptamine
detn	detention
dets	let it be given and labeled *(detur et signatur)*
dev	develop, development • deviate, deviation
DEV	duck embryo vaccine
devel	develop, development
DF	decayed and filled (teeth) • degrees of freedom (a statistical parameter) • dorsiflexion • dry gas phase fractional concentration
DFA	diet for age • direct fluorescent antibody (technique)
DFDD	difluorodiphenyldichloroethane
DFDT	difluorodiphenyltrichloroethane
DFMC	daily fetal movement count
DFO	deferoxamine (desferrioxamine)
DFP	disopropylfluorophosphate
DFR	dialysate filtration rate
DFS	disease-free survival
DFT$_4$	dialyzable free thyroxine 4
DFU	dead fetus in utero
dg	decigram
DG	deoxyglucose • diagnose, diagnosis, diagnostic • diglyceride

DGI	disseminated gonococcal infection
dgm	decigram
dGMP	deoxyguanosine monophosphate (deoxyguanylate)
DGVB	dextrose, gelatin, Veronal buffer
DH	delayed hypersensitivity • dermatitis herpetiformis • diffuse and histiocytic
DHA	dehydroepiandrosterone • dihydroxyacetone
DHE	dihydroergotamine
DHEA	dehydropiandrosterone
DHEAS	dehydroepiandrosterone sulfate
DHEW	Department of Health, Education and Welfare
DHF	dengue hemorrhagic fever
DHFR	dihydrofolate reductase
DHHS	Department of Health and Human Services
DHL	diffuse histiocytic lymphoma
DHO	deuterium hydrogen oxide
DHPR	dihydropteridine reductase
DHS	Department of Health Services • direct health service • duration of hospital stay
DHSM	dihydrostreptomycin
DHSQ	Division of Health Standards and Quality
DHT	dihydrotachysterol • dihydrotestosterone
DHy	Doctor of Hygiene
Di	Diego blood group
DI	deterioration index • diabetes insipidus • disability insurance • distoincisal • double indemnity
dia	diameter, diatherm
diab	diabetes, diabetic
diag	diagnosis, diagnostic • diagonal • diagram
diam	diameter

diath	diathermy
DIB	disability insurance benefit
DIC	diffuse intravascular coagulation • drug information center
DIDMOAD	diabetes insipidus, diabetes mellitus, optic atrophy, deafness
dieb alt	on alternate days (*diebus alternis*)
dieb tert	every third day (*diebus tertiis*)
dif	differential blood count • differential leukocyte count
DIF	diffuse interstitial fibrosis • direct immunofluorescence
Diff	difference, different • differential • differential blood count, differential leukocyte count
diff diag	differential diagnosis
DIFP	diisopropyl fluorophosphonate
dig	digitalis
Dig	digitalis
dil	dilute, diluted, dilution
dilat	dilate, dilated, dilation, dilatation
DILD	diffuse infiltrative lung disease
dilut	dilute, diluted, dilution
dim	dimension, diminish, diminutive
DIM	one-half (*dimidius*)
dIMP	deoxyinosine monophosphate (deoxyinosinate)
d in p aeq	divide into equal parts (*divide in partes aequales*)
diopt	diopter
DIP	desquamative interstitial pneumonia • distal interphalangeal
DIPC	diffuse interstitial pulmonary calcification
DIPF	diisopropylphosphofluoridate
diph	diphtheria

DIPJ	distal interphalangeal joint
dir	direct
dis	disabled, disease, distance
disc	discontinue
disch	discharge, discharge
DISH	diffuse idiopathic skeletal hyperostosis
disloc	dislocate, dislocation
disp	dispense, dispensary
dissd	dissolved
dissem	disseminate, disseminated, dissemination
dist	distal • distill, distilled • distribute, distribution • disturbance
distill	distillation
DIT	diiodotyrosine
div	divergence • divide, division • divorced
DJD	degenerative joint disease
DKA	diabetic ketoacidosis
dkg	dekagram
dkl	dekaliter
dkm	dekameter
DKS	deoxyketosteroids
dl	deciliter
DL	danger list • diffusing capacity of the lung • direct laryngoscopy • distolingual • Donath-Landsteiner (test)
DLa	distolabial
DLaI	distolabioincisal
DLaP	distolabiopulpal
DLB	diffuse and lymphoblastic
DLCO	diffusing capacity of the lung

DLCO-SB	single-breath diffusing capacity of the lung for carbon monoxide
DLE	discoid lupus erythematosus • disseminated lupus erythematosus
DLI	distolinguoincisal
dm	decimeter
DM	diabetes mellitus • diastolic murmur • dopamine • double minute • membrane-diffusing capacity
DMA	dimethyladenosine • directed memory access
DMABA	dimethylaminobenzaldehyde
DMARD	disease-modifying antirheumatic drug
DMAT	disaster medical assistance team
DMCT	demethylchlortetracycline
DMD	Doctor of Dental Medicine *(Dentariae Medicinae Doctor)*
DME	direct medical education • Director of Medical Education • durable medical equipment
DMERC	durable medical equipment regional carriers
DMF	decayed, missing, or filled (teeth)
DMFS	decayed, missing or filled surfaces
DMHS	Department of Mental Health Services
DMI	diaphragmatic myocardial infarction
DMM	dimethylmyleran
DMN	dimethylnitrosamine
DMNA	dimethylnitrosamine
DMO	dimethyloxazolidinedione
DMOC	diabetes mellitus out of control
DMOOC	diabetes mellitus out of control
DMP	dimethylphosphate • dimethylphthalate
DMPA	depomedroxyprogesterone acetate

DMS	delayed muscle soreness • dermatomyositis • Director of Medical Services
DMSA	dimercaptosuccinic acid
DMSO	dimethylsulfoxide
DMT	dimethyltryptamine (hallucinogenic drug)
DN	dicrotic notch
D/N	dextrose-nitrogen ratio
DNA	deoxyribonucleic acid
DNase	deoxyribonuclease
DNB	dinitrobenzene
DNCB	dinitrochlorobenzene
DNE	Director of Nursing Education
DNFB	dinitrofluorbenzene
DNI	do not intubate
DNP	deoxyribonucleoprotein • dinitrophenyl
DNPH	dinitrophenylhydrazine
DNPM	dinitrophenylmorphine
DNR	daunorubicin • do not report • do not resuscitate
DNS	deviated nasal septum • Director of Nursing Service • dysplastic nevus syndrome
D5/NS	5% dextrose in normal saline
DO	diamine oxidase • dissolved oxygen • disto-occlusal • Doctor of Osteopathy • doctor's orders
DOA	date of admission • dead on arrival
DOB	date of birth • doctor's order book
doc	diabetes out of control • document, documentation
DOC	deoxycholate • deoxycorticosterone • diabetes out of control • drug of choice
DOCA	deoxycorticosterone acetate
DOC-SR	deoxycorticosterone secretion rate

DOE	desoxyephedrine • dyspnea on exertion
DOES	disorders of excessive somnolence
dom	dominant
DOM	dimethoxymethylamphetamine
DON	Director of Nurses
DOOC	diabetes out of control
DOPA	dihydroxyphenylalanine
DOPAC	dihydroxyphenylacetic acid
DOPS	diffuse obstructive pulmonary syndrome
dos	dose, dosage
DOS	day of surgery
DOT	died on (operating) table
DOU	Definitive Observation Unit
doz	dozen
DP	data processing • deep pulse, dementia praecox • diastolic pressure • diffusion pressure • digestible protein • diphosgene • disopyramide phosphate • displaced person • distal pancreatectomy • distopulpal • Doctor of Pharmacy • Doctor of Podiatry • donor's plasma • dorsalis pedis • dyspnea
DPA	diphenylamine
DPAHC	Durable Power of Attorney for Health Care
DPD	diffuse pulmonary disease
DPDA	phosphorodiamidic anhydride
DPDL	diffuse poorly differentiated lymphocytic
DPDT	double-pole, double-throw (switch)
DPG	diphosphoglycerate • displacement placentogram
DPH	Department of Public Health • diphenylhydantoin • Diploma in Public Health • Doctor of Public Health
dpm	disintegrations per minute

DPM	Doctor of Podiatric Medicine
DPN	diphosphopyridine nucleotide
DPNH	diphosphopyridine nucleotide, reduced form
DPO	designated provider organization
DPP	documented poor prognosis
dps	disintegrations per second
DPST	double-pole, single-throw (switch)
DPT	diphtheria, pertussis and tetanus toxoid • diphtheria toxoid-pertussis vaccine-tetanus toxoid immunization • Demerol, Phenergan and Thorazine
DPTI	diastolic pressure-time index
DQ	deterioration quotient • developmental quotient
dr	dram • dressing
Dr	doctor
DR	degeneration reaction • delivery room • diabetic retinopathy • diagnostic radiology • diurnal rhythm • dorsal root
DRA	despite resuscitation attempts
DRF	daily replacement factor
DRG	Diagnosis Related Group
D(Rh$_0$)	blood antigen
drng	drainage
DRQ	discomfort relief quotient
DRS	data retrieval system
drsg	dressing
DRTC	Diabetes Research and Training Center

DS	dead (air) space • dehydroepiandrosterone sulfate • depolarizing shift • density standard • desynchronized sleep • dextran sulfate • dextrose in saline • dilute strength • dioptic strength • Doctor of Science • donor's serum • double-stranded • double-strength • Down syndrome • duration of systole
D-S	Doerfler-Stewart (test)
DSA	digital subtraction angiography
DSAP	disseminated superficial actinic porokeratosis
DSB	drug-seeking behavior
DSC	Doctor of Surgical Chiropody
DSCG	disodium cromoglycate
DSD	dry sterile dressing
dsg	dressing
DSH	deliberate self-harm • disproportionate share hospital
DSI	drug-seeking index
DSM	Diagnostic and Statistical Manual of Mental Disorders
DSS	dengue shock syndrome
DST	desensitization test • dexamethasone suppression test
D-stix	dextrostix
DSVP	downstream venous pressure
Dt	duration of tetany
DT	delirium tremens • Dietetic Services • diphtheria and tetanus toxoids • distance test • doubling time (of tumor size) • duration of tetany
DTBC	d-tubocurarine
dtd	give of such a dose *(datur talis dosis)*
DTIC	dacarbazine
DTM	dermatophyte test medium
DTN	diphtheria toxin, normal
DTNB	dithiobisnitrobenzoic acid

DTP	diphtheria toxoid-tetanus toxoid-pertussis vaccine immunization • distal tingling on percussion
DTPA	diethylenetriamine penta-acetic acid
DTR	deep tendon reflex
DTS	discrete time sample
DTX	detoxification
DU	deoxyuridine • diagnosis undetermined • diffuse and undifferentiated • dog unit • duodenal ulcer
DUB	dysfunctional uterine bleeding
DUG	drug use guidelines
DUI	driving under the influence
DUL	diffuse undifferentiated lymphoma
dUMP	deoxyuridine monophosphate (deoxyuridylate)
dup	duplicate, duplication
DUR	Drug Usage Review
dur dolor	while the pain lasts (*durante dolore*)
DUS	Doppler Ultrasound Stethoscope
dv	double vision
DV	dependent variable • dilute volume • direct vision • distance vision • double vibration
D&V	diarrhea and vomiting
DVA	duration of voluntary apnea (test)
DVI	Digital Vascular Imaging
DVM	Doctor of Veterinary Medicine
DVMS	Doctor of Veterinary Medicine and Surgery
DVS	Doctor of Veterinary Science • Doctor of Veterinary Surgery
DVT	deep venous thrombus
DVVC	direct visualization of vocal cords
DW	distilled water • dry weight

D/W	dextrose in water
D₅W	5% dextrose in water
DWDL	diffuse, well-differentiated, lymphocytic
Dx	diagnosis
DX	dextran
DXM	dexamethasone
DXR	deep x-ray
DXRT	deep x-ray therapy
DXT	deep x-ray therapy
Dy	dysprosium
DZ	dizygotic, dizygous

E

e	base of natural-logarithm system (approximately 2.71828) • electric charge • electron • from *(ex)*
E	electrode potential • electromotive force • emmetropia • enema • energy • enzyme • epidural • epinephrine • erythrocyte • *Escherichia* • experimenter • expired (gas) • extinction coefficient • eye
E₁	estrone
E₂	estradiol
E₃	estriol
ea	each
EA	early antigen • educational age • electroanesthesia • environmental assessment • erythrocyte antibody
E&A	evaluate and advise
EAA	essential amino acid
EAB	extra-anatomic bypass
EAC	erythrocyte antibody complement • external auditory canal
EACA	epsilon-aminocaproic acid
EACD	eczematous allergic contact dermatitis
ead	the same *(eadem)*
EAD	early after-depolarization
EAE	experimental allergic encephalomyelitis
EAHF	eczema, asthma, hay fever
EAI	electronically assisted instruction
EAL	electronic artificial larynx

EAM	external acoustic meatus
EAMG	experimental allergic myasthenia gravis
EAN	experimental allergic rhinitis
EANG	epidemic acute nonbacterial gastroenteritis
EAP	employee assistance program • epiallopregnanolone
EaR	reaction of degeneration *(Entartungs Reaktion)*
EB	elementary body • Epstein-Barr virus
EBAA	Eye Bank Association of America
EBBS	equal bilateral breath sounds
EBCDIC	extended binary-coded decimal interchange code
EBF	erythroblastosis fetalis
EBI	emetine bismuth iodine
EBL	estimated blood loss
EBM	expressed breast milk
EBNA	Epstein-Barr virus nuclear antigen
EBP	epidural blood patch • estradiol-binding protein
EBS	electric brain stimulator
EBV	Epstein-Barr virus
EC	electron capture • emergency center • enteric-coated • entrance complaint • Enzyme Commission • expiratory center • extracellular compartment
E-C	ether-chloroform
E/C	estriol-creatinine ratio
ECA	electrocardioanalyzer • epidemiological catchment area
ECBO	enteric cytopathogenic bovine orphan (virus)
ECC	emergency cardiac care • external cardiac compression • extracorporeal circulation
ECCE	extracapsular cataract extraction
ECD	electron-capture detector

ECF	extended-care facility • extracellular fluid
ECF-A	eosinophilic chemotactic factor of anaphylaxis
ECFMG	Educational Council for Foreign Medical Graduates
ECG	electrocardiogram, electrocardiography
echo	echoencephalogram, echoencephalography
Echo	echocardiogram
ECHO	electronic computing health oriented • enteric cytopathogenic human orphan (virus)
ECI	extracorporeal irradiation
eclec	eclectic
ECM	egg crate mattress • erythema chronicum migrans • extracellular matrix
ECMO	enteric cytopathogenic monkey orphan (virus)
ECOG	Eastern Cooperative Oncology Group
E coli	*Escherichia coli*
econ	economic
ECP	electronic claims processing • external counter-pulsation
ECPO	enteric cytopathogenic porcine orphan (virus)
ECPOG	electrochemical potential gradient
ECS	electrocerebral silence • electroconvulsive shock • electronic claims submission
ECSO	enteric cytopathogenic swine orphan (virus)
ECT	electroconvulsive therapy • enteric-coated tablet
ECV	extracellular volume
ECW	extracellular water
ed	editor
ED	effective dose • emergency department • epidural • erythema dose
ED$_{50}$	median effective dose
EDB	early dry breakfast • ethylene dibromide

EDC	effective dynamic compliance • estimated date of confinement
ED&C	electrodesiccation and curettage
Ed.D.	Doctor of Education
EDD	end-diastolic dimension • estimated discharge date • expected date of delivery
edent	edentulous
edit	editorial
EDN	electrodesiccation
EDP	electronic data processing • emergency department physician • end diastolic pressure
EDR	effective direct radiation • electrodermal response • expected death rate
EDS	Ehlers-Danlos syndrome • extended data stream
EDTA	edetate disodium • edetic acid • ethylene-diaminetetra-acetic acid
educ	education
EDV	end-diastolic volume
EDx	electrodiagnosis
EE	embryo extract • equine encephalitis • eye and ear
EEC	enteropathogenic *E. coli*
EEE	eastern equine encephalomyelitis
EEG	electroencephalogram, electroencephalography
EENT	eye, ear, nose and throat
EEOC	Equal Employment Opportunity Commission
EEP	end-expiratory pressure
EERP	extended endocardial resection procedure
EES	erythromycin ethylsuccinate
EF	ejection fraction • elongation factor • equivalent focus • erythroblastosis fetalis • erythrocytic fragmentation • exophthalmic factor • extended-field (radiotherapy) • extrinsic factor

EFA	Epilepsy Foundation of America • essential fatty acids
EFAD	essential fatty acid deficiency
EFE	endocardial fibroelastosis
eff	effect(s), effective • efferent • efficient
EFM	electronic fetal monitoring
EFP	effective filtration pressure
EFR	effective filtration rate
eg	for example *(exempli gratia)*
EGA	estimated gestational age
EGC	epithelioid A globoid cells
EGD	esophagogastroduodenoscopy
EGF	epidermal growth factor
EGFR	epidermal growth factor receptor
EGG	electrogastrogram
EGHP	employer group health plan
EGOT	erythrocyte glutamic oxaloacetic transaminase
EGR	erythrocyte glutathione reductase
EGTA	esophageal gastric tube airway
eH	oxidation-reduction potential
E$_h$	oxidation-reduction potential
EH	enlarged heart • essential hypertension
E&H	environment and heredity
EHBF	estimated hepatic blood flow • extrahepatic blood flow
EHBFF	extrahepatic blood flow factor
EHC	enterohepatic circulation • enterohepatic clearance
EHDP	disodium etidronate • ethane hydroxydiphosphate
EHF	exophthalmos-hyperthyroid factor

EHH	esophageal hiatal hernia
EHIP	employee health insurance plan
EHL	effective half-life
EHPT	Eddy hot plate test
EHSDS	experimental health services delivery system
EIA	enzyme immunoassay • exercise-induced asthma
EIS	Epidemic Intelligence Service
EIT	erythrocyte iron turnover
EJ	elbow jerk
ejusd	of the same *(ejusdem)*
EKC	epidemic keratoconjunctivitis
EKG	electrocardiogram
EKY	electrokymogram
EL	effective level • exercise limit
E-L	Eaton-Lambert syndrome
elb	elbow
ELB	early light breakfast
elect	electric, electricity
ELF	elective low forceps (delivery)
ELG	eligible
ELISA	enzyme-linked immunosorbent assay
elix	elixir
ELM	Early Language Milestone Scale
ELT	euglobulin lysis time
elytes	electrolytes
em	electromagnetic
EM	effective masking • electron microscope • emergency medicine • emmetropia
E-M	Embden-Meyerhof (glycolytic pathway)

E&M	endocrine and metabolic
EMA	emergency medical attendant
Emb	embryo, embryology
EMB	eosin methylene blue • ethambutol
EMC	encephalomyocarditis
EMCRO	Experimental Medical Care Review Organization
emer	emergency
emf	electromotive force
EMF	electromotive force • endomyocardial fibrosis • erythrocyte maturation factor
EMG	electromyogram, electromyography • exophthalmos, macroglossia, and gigantism
EMGN	extra-membranous glomerulonephritis
EMI	electromagnetic interference
EMIC	emergency maternity and infant care
EMIT	enzyme-multiplied immunoassay technique
emot	emotion, emotional
emp	as directed *(ex modo praescripto)* • plaster *(emplastrum)*
EMPEP	erythrocyte membrane protein electrophoretic pattern
EMR	electromagnetic radiation
EMS	early morning specimen • Emergency Medical Service • Emergency Medical System
EMT	emergency medical technician • emergency medical treatment
emu	electromagnetic unit
emul	emulsion
en	enema
EN	enteral nutrition • erythema nodosum
ENA	extractable nuclear antigen
enem	enema

ENG	electronystagmography
enl	enlarged
ENL	erythema nodosum leprosum
ENNS	Early Neonatal Neurobehavior Scale
ENT	ear, nose and throat
environ	environment, environmental
enz	enzyme
EO	ethylene oxide
EOA	Equal Opportunity Act • esophageal obturator airway • examination, opinion and advice
EOB	explanation of benefits
EOC	episode of care
eod	every other day
EOD	environmental and occupational disorders
EOE	Equal Opportunity Employer
EOF	end of field • end of file
EOG	electro-oculogram, electro-oculography
EOM	extraocular movement • extraocular muscles
EOMB	explanation of medical benefits
EOP	endogenous opioid peptides
eos	eosinophil
EOS	eligibility on-site
EP	ectopic pregnancy • electrophoresis • emergency physician • endogenous pyrogen • erythrocyte protoporphyrin • esophoria
EPA	Environmental Protection Agency • erect posteroanterior
EPC	epilepsia partialis continua
EPCG	endoscopic pancreatocholangiography
EPEA	expense per equivalent admission

EPEC	enteropathogenic *E. coli*
EPF	exophthalmos-producing factor
EPI	epinephrine
epil	epilepsy
epis	episiotomy
EPITH	epithelium, epithelial
EPO	exclusive provider organization
EPP	equal pressure point • erythropoietic protoporphyria
EPPS	Edwards Personal Preference Schedule
EPR	electron paramagnetic resonance • electrophrenic respiration
EPS	elastosis perforans serpiginosa • exophthalmos-producing substance • expressed prostate secretions • extrapyramidal symptoms • extrapyramidal syndrome
EPSDT	early and periodic screening, diagnosis and treatment
EPSE	extrapyramidal side effects
EPSP	excitatory postsynaptic potential
EPTS	existed prior to service
eq	equal • equation • equilibrium • equivalent
EQ	educational quotient
EQA	external quality assessment
equilib	equilibrium
equip	equipment
equiv	equivalent
Er	erbium
ER	emergency room • endoplasmic reticulum • equivalent roentgen • estradiol receptor • estrogen receptor • evoked response • extended release • external resistance • external rotation
ERA	electric response audiometry • evoked response audiometry

ERBF	effective renal blood flow
ERC	endoscopic retrograde cholangiography
ERCP	endoscopic retrograde cannulization of pancreas • endoscopic retrograde cholangio- pancreatography
ERD	evoked response detector
erf	error function
ERF	Education and Research Foundation (AMA)
erg	energy unit
ERG	electrolyte replacement with glucose • electroretinogram, electroretinography
ERIA	electroradio-immuno assay
ERO	external review organization
ERP	early receptor potential • effective refractory period • emergency room physician • endoscopic retrograde pancreatography • estrogen receptor protein
ERPF	effective renal plasma flow
ERT	estrogen replacement therapy
ERV	expiratory reserve volume
Ery	*Erysipelothrix*
Es	einsteinium • electrical stimulation • estriol
ES	Emergency Service • end stage • end-to-side
ESB	electrical stimulation of the brain
Esch	*Escherichia*
ESD	end-systolic dimension • esophagus, stomach and duodenum
ESE	electrostatic unit *(electrostatische Einheit)*
ESF	erythropoietic-stimulating factor
ESG	electrospinogram • estrogen
ESN	educationally subnormal
ESO	esophagus

esp	especially
ESP	Economic Stabilization Program • electrosensitive point • end systolic pressure • extrasensory perception
ESR	electron spin resonance • erythrocyte sedimentation rate
ESRD	end-stage renal disease
ess	essential, essentially
ESS	empty sella syndrome
est	estimated
EST	electroshock therapy
esu	electrostatic unit
ESU	electrostatic unit • electrosurgical unit
ESV	end-systolic volume
ESWL	extracorporeal shock wave lithotripsy
et	and *(et)* • etiology
Et	ethyl
ET	educational therapy • endotracheal • endotracheal tube • enterostomal therapy, therapist • esotropia, esotropic • eustachian tube • exercise treadmill
ETA	endotracheal aspirates • ethionamide
et al	and others *(et alii)*
E$_T$CO$_2$	end-tidal carbon dioxide concentration
ETD	estimated time of death
ETEC	enterotoxigenic *Escherichia coli*
ETF	electron-transferring flavoprotein
eth	ether
ETI	ejective time index
etiol	etiology
EtO	ethylene oxide

Et₂O	ether
ETO	estimated time of ovulation
ETOH	ethyl alcohol
ETP	elective termination of pregnancy
ETR	effective thyroxine ratio
ETT	endotracheal tube • exercise tolerance test • exercise treadmill test
Eu	europium
EUA	examination under anesthesia
EUCD	emotionally unstable character disorder
ev	electron-volt • eversion
eV	electron-volt
EV	extravascular
evac	evacuated, evacuation
eval	evaluate, evaluation
evap	evaporate, evaporation
EVR	evoked visual response
EW	emergency ward
EWL	evaporative water loss
Ex	examination • exercise • former
exam	examination, examiner
exc	except • excision
exec	executive
exhib	let it be given *(exhibeatur)*
exist	existing
exp	expected • expired • exponent
exper	experimental
expir	expiration, expiratory
expn	expression

exptl	experimental
ext	extensor • exterior • external • extract, extraction • extremity, extremities • spread (extend)
Ext FHR	external fetal heart rate (monitoring)
ext fl	fluid extract
extrap	extrapolate, extrapolation
EY	ophthalmologic disease

F

f	frequency
F	brother *(frater)* • facies • Fahrenheit • failure • family • farad, farady • father • fecal • fellow • female • fetal • field (visual) • fluorine • flutter wave • foot • force • formula, formulary • fractional concentration • French (catheter size) • function • fusion beat • make *(fac)* • son *(filus)*
FA	Family Anonymous • Fanconi's anemia • fatty acid • femoral artery • fertilization antigen • field ambulance • filterable agent • filtered air • first aid • fluorescent antibody • folic acid • forearm • fortified aqueous (solution) • fusaric acid
FAAN	Fellow of the American Academy of Nursing
FAB	French-American-British (Cooperative Group, classification) • functional arm brace
FAC	fluorouracil, Adriamycin, cyclophosphamide • free-standing ambulatory care
FACA	Fellow of the American College of Anesthesiologists
FACD	Fellow of the American College of Dentists
FACHA	Fellow of the American College of Hospital Administrators
FACNM	Fellow of the American College of Nuclear Medicine
FACOG	Fellow of the American College of Obstetrics and Gynecology
FACP	Fellow of the American College of Physicians
FACSM	Fellow of the American College of Sports Medicine
FAD	flavin adenine dinucleotide
FADH$_2$	flavin adenine dinucleotide, reduced form

FAI	functional aerobic impairment
fam	family
FAMA	Fellow of the American Medical Association • fluorescent antibody membrane antigen (test)
fam doc	family doctor
FAMLIES	Financial support, Advocacy, Medical management, Love, Information, Education, Structural support
FANA	fluorescent antinuclear antibody
FAOTA	Fellow of the American Occupational Therapy Association
FAP	familial adenomatous polyposis
FAPHA	Fellow of the American Public Health Association
far	farad, faradic
FAR	flight aptitude rating
F^{AR}	immediate good function followed by accelerated rejection
FAS	fetal alcohol syndrome • Financial Analysis Service
FASA	Freestanding Ambulatory Surgery Association
fasc	bundle (*fasciculus*)
FASC	freestanding ambulatory surgery center
FAT	fluorescent antibody test
FB	fingerbreadth • foreign body
FBCOD	foreign body cornea left eye
FBCOS	foreign body cornea right eye
FBG	fasting blood glucose
FBI	flossing, brushing, irrigation
FBM	fetal breathing movements
FBP	fibrin breakdown products • fructose biphosphate
FBS	fasting blood sugar • feedback signal • feedback system • fetal bovine serum
FBU	fingers below umbilicus

Fc	foot-candle
FC	finger count • fluorocytosine • Foley catheter • functional class
F/C	fever and chills
FCC	follicular center cell • fracture - compound, comminuted
FCP	final common pathway
FCSA	Federal Controlled Substances Act
FD	family doctor • fatal dose • fibrinogen derivative • fixed and dilated • focal distance • forceps delivery • freeze-dried
FD$_{50}$	median fatal dose
F/D	fracture dislocation
FDA	Food and Drug Administration
FD&C Act	Food, Drug and Cosmetic Act
FDF	fast death factor
fdg	feeding
FDG	fluoro-18-deoxyglucose
FDIU	fetal death in utero
FDNB	fluorodinitrobenzene
FDP	fibrin degradation products
FDRA	food and drug reactions and anaphylaxis
Fe	iron *(ferrum)*
FE	fatty ester • fetal erythroblastosis
feb dur	while the fever lasts *(febre durante)*
FEC	freestanding emergency center
FECG	fetal electrocardiogram
FeCl$_3$	ferric chloride
FeCN	ferricyanide
FECT	fibro-elastic connective tissue

FEEG	fetal electroencephalogram
FEF	forced expiratory flow
FEHBP	Federal Employees Health Benefits Plan
FEKG	fetal electrocardiogram
FEL	familial erythrophagocytic lymphohistiocytosis
FELV	feline leukemia virus
fem	female • thigh (*femoris*)
FEP	free erythrocyte protoporphyrin
ferv	boiling (*fervens*)
FES	functional electrical stimulation
FETI	fluorescence energy transfer immunoassay
Fe/TIBC	iron saturation of serum transferrin
FEV	forced expiratory volume
FEV$_1$	one-second forced expiratory volume
FEV$_1$/FVC	ratio of one-second forced expiratory volume to forced vital capacity
ff	following • force fluids
FF	fat-free • filtration fraction • fixing fluid • flat feet • force fluids • foster father • fresh frozen • fundus firm
FFA	female-female adaptor • free fatty acid
FFC	free from chlorine
FFD	focus-to-film distance (x-ray)
FFDW	fat-free dry weight
FFF	fair, fat and forty
FFI	Family Functioning Index • free from infection
FFP	Federal Financial Participation • fresh frozen plasma
FFS	fat-free supper • fee-for-service • flexible fiberoptic sigmoidoscopy
FFT	flicker fusion threshold

FFWW	fat-free wet weight
fg	femtogram
FGT	female genital tract
FH	family history • fetal heart • Frankfort horizontal (plane of the skull)
FH₄	folacin
FHC	family health center
FHMI	family history of mental illness
FHNH	fetal heart not heard
FHR	fetal heart rate
FHS	fetal heart sounds
FHT	fetal heart tones
FHVP	free hepatic venous pressure
FHx	family history
FI	fiscal intermediary
FIA	fluorescence immunoassay • Freedom of Information Act
fib	fibrillation
FICA	Federal Insurance Contribution Act
FICD	Fellow of the International College of Dentists
FICS	Fellow of the International College of Surgeons
FID	flame-ionization detector
FIF	formaldehyde-induced fluorescence
fig	figure
FIGLU	formiminoglutamic acid
FIGO	International Federation of Obstetricians and Gynecologists
FIH	fat-induced hyperglycemia
filt	filter
FIN	fine intestinal needle

FiO₂	fractional inspiratory oxygen
FIO₂	forced inspiratory oxygen
fist	fistula
FIT	Food Intolerance Testing
FITC	fluorescein isothiocyanate, conjugated
FJRM	full joint range of motion
fl	flexion • fluid
FL	focal length
fla	let it be done according to the rule (*fiat lege artis*)
fld	field • fluid
fl dr	fluid dram
flex	flexion
FLEX	Federation Licensing Examination
flor	flowers
fl oz	fluid ounce
Fluo	fluothane
fluores	fluorescence, fluorescent
fm	make a mixture (*fiat mistura*)
Fm	fermium
FM	fetal movements • flavin mononucleotide • frequency modulation
FMC	Foundation for Medical Care
FMD	fibromuscular dysplasia • foot and mouth disease
FME	full-mouth extraction
fMet	formylmethionine
FMF	familial Mediterranean fever
FMG	foreign medical graduate
FMH	fat-mobilizing hormone • fetal-maternal hemorrhage
FML	fluorometholone

FMN	flavin mononucleotide
FMNH$_2$	flavin mononucleotide, reduced form
FMP	first menstrual period
FMR	Friend-Moloney-Rauscher (virus)
FMS	false memory syndrome • fat-mobilizing substance • full mouth series
FMX	full-mouth x-rays
fn	function
FN	false-negative • finger to nose (coordination test)
FNA(C)	fine needle aspiration (cytology)
FNH	focal nodular hyperplasia
fn p	fusion point
FNP	Family Nurse Practitioner
FNTC	fine needle transhepatic cholangiography
FO	focus out • foramen ovale • fronto-occipital
FOB	fecal occult blood • fiberoptic bronchoscopy • foot of bed
FOIA	Freedom of Information Act
FOM	figure of merit (measure of diagnostic value per radionuclide radiation dose)
for	foreign
FOR	forensic
fort	strong (*fortis*)
FORTRAN	Formula Translation
found	foundation
fp	freezing point
FP	false-positive • family physician • family planning • flat plate • family practice • family practitioner • Federation Proceedings • flavin phosphate • fluid pressure • frozen plasma

FPC	family practice center • fish protein concentrate • frozen packed cells
FPG	fasting plasma glucose
FPHx	family psychiatric history
FPIA	fluorescence polarization immunoassay
fpm	feet per minute
FPM	filter paper microscopic (test)
FPMP	Federal Preventive Medicine Program
fps	feet per second • foot-pound-second (system)
FPS	foot-pound-second (system)
fr	from
Fr	francium
FR	flocculation reaction • French (catheter size)
F&R	force and rhythm
FRA	fluorescent rabies antibody (test) • right frontoanterior
frac	fracture
fract dos	in divided doses (*fracta dosi*)
frag	fragile • fragment
FRC	frozen red cells • functional residual capacity
FRCP	Fellow of the Royal College of Physicians
FRCS	Fellow of the Royal College of Surgeons
freq	frequency
FRF	follicle-stimulating hormone-releasing factor
FRH	follicle-stimulating hormone-releasing hormone
Fried	Friedman's test
frig	refrigerator
FRJM	full-range joint movement
FROM	full range of motion

FRS	Fellow of the Royal Society • first rank symptoms (Schneider's)
FRT	full recovery time
FRV	functional residual volume
FS	factor of safety • fracture - simple • forearm supinated • frozen section • full soft • full strength
FSB	fetal scalp blood
FSBG	finger-stick blood gas
FSC	fracture - simple, comminuted
FSD	focus-to-skin distance (x-ray)
FSF	fibrin-stabilizing factor
FSGS	focal segmental glomerulosclerosis
FSH	follicle-stimulating hormone
FSH-RF	follicle-stimulating hormone-releasing factor
FSH-RH	follicle-stimulating hormone-releasing hormone
FSI	foam stability index
FSP	fibrin split products
ft	foot • let it be made (*fiat*)
ft^2	square foot
ft^3	cubic foot
Ft	ferritin
FT	full-term
FT$_3$	free triiodothyronine
FT$_4$	free thyroxine
FTA	fluorescent treponemal antibody
FTA-ABS	fluorescent treponemal antibody absorption (test)
F-TAG	fast-binding target-attaching globulin
FTBD	full-term born dead
ft c	foot-candle

FTC	Federal Trade Commission
FTE	full-time employee • full-time equivalent
FTI	free thyroxine index
ft lb	foot-pound
FTND	full term normal delivery
FTP	failure to progress
FTSG	full-thickness skin graft
FTT	failure to thrive
FU	fat unit • fecal urobilinogen • Finsen unit • fluorouracil • follow-up • fractional analysis
FU-I, FU-II	first, second set of follow-up data
FUB	functional uterine bleeding
FUDR	fluorodeoxyuridine
func	function, functional
FUO	fever of undetermined origin • fever of unknown origin
fu p	fusion point
FUT	fibrinogen uptake test
FV	femoral vein
FVC	false vocal cord • forced vital capacity • functional vital capacity
FWB	full-weight-bearing
FWHM	full width at half maximum
FWR	Felix-Weil reaction
FWW	front-wheel walker
Fx	fracture • friction
FY	fiscal year
FYI	for your information
FZ	focal zone • frozen section

G

g	gas • grain • gram
G	gastrin • gauge • gauss • gender • giga- • gingival • glucose • good • gram • gravid, gravida • gravity • Greek • guanine • guanosine • Newtonian constant of gravitation
Ga	gallium
GA	gastric analysis • general anesthesia • general assistance • gingivoaxial
GABA	gamma-aminobutyric acid
GAD	glutamic acid decarboxylase
GAF	global assessment of functioning
GAG	glycosaminoglycan
gal	galactose • gallon
gal/min	gallons per minute
GALT	gut-associated lymphoid tissue
galv	galvanic
gang	ganglion, ganglionic
garg	gargle
GAS	general adaptation syndrome • generalized arteriosclerosis • Global Assessment Scale • Group A streptococcus
Gas Anal F&T	gas analysis, free and total
GASCVD	generalized arteriosclerotic cardiovascular disease
GASP	Group Against Smokers' Pollution
gastroc	gastrocnemius
GAW	airway conductance

GB	gallbladder • Guillain-Barré (syndrome)
GBA	gingivobuccoaxial
GBBS	group B beta-hemolytic streptococcus
GBM	glomerular basement membrane
GBS	gallbladder series • group B streptococcus • Guillain-Barré syndrome
GC	gas chromatography • gastrointestinal catastrophe • glucocorticoid • gonococcus, gonococcal • guanine-cytosine
GCA	giant-cell arteritis
g-cal	gram calorie (small calorie)
GCFT	gonorrhea complement fixation test
g-cm	gram-centimeter
GCS	general clinical service • Glasgow coma scale
Gd	gadolinium
GD	given dose • Graves' disease
GDM	gestational diabetes mellitus
GDP	guanosine diphosphate
GDTP	goal-directed therapy program
Ge	germanium
GE	gastroenterology
GEF	gonadotrophin enhancing factor
gen	general • genus
geom	geometric
GEP	gastroenteropancreatic (endocrine system)
GER	gastroesophageal reflux
GERD	gastroesophageal reflux disease
GET	gastric emptying time
GF	gastric fistula • germ-free • girlfriend • globule fibril • glomerular filtration • grandfather • growth fraction

GFR	glomerular filtration rate
GG	Gamma globulin • glyceryl guaiacolate
GGE	generalized glandular enlargement
GGT	gamma-glutamyltransferase • gamma-glutamyltranspeptidase
GGTP	gamma-glutamyltranspeptidase
GH	general hospital • growth hormone
GHA	Group Health Association
GHAA	Group Health Association of America
GHb	glycosylated hemoglobin
GHB	glycosylated hemoglobin
GHBP	growth hormone-binding protein
GHPP	Genetically Handicapped Persons Program
GHQ	general health questionnaire
GHRF	growth hormone-releasing factor
GHRH	growth hormone-releasing hormone
GHRIF	growth hormone release-inhibiting factor
GI	gastrointestinal • Gingival Index • globin insulin • glomerular index • growth-inhibiting
GIBF	gastrointestinal bacterial flora
GIFT	gamete intra-Fallopian transfer
GIGO	garbage in, garbage out (computer data)
GIK	glucose-insulin-potassium
GII	gastrointestinal infection
GIP	gastric inhibitory peptide • gastric inhibitory polypeptide
GIS	gastrointestinal series
GIT	gastrointestinal tract
GITT	glucose-insulin tolerance test
GIV	gastrointestinal virus

GIX	an insecticidal compound
GK	galactokinase
gl	gland, glands
GL	greatest length
GLA	gingivolinguoaxial
glc	glaucoma
GLC	gas-liquid chromatography
Gln	glutamine
Glob	globular • globulin
glu	glucose
Glu	glutamate
Gluc	glucose
glucur	glucuronide
glu ox	glucose oxidase
glut max	gluteus maximus
glut med	gluteus medius
GLV	Gross leukemia virus
Gly	glycine
glyc	glycerin
gm	gram
Gm	gram
GM	grand mal (epilepsy) • grandmother
GMC	General Medical Council
gm cal	gram calorie (small calorie)
GMENAC	Graduate Medical Education National Advisory Committee
GMK	green monkey kidney
GML	glabellomeatal line
gm-m	gram-meter

GMP	guanosine monophosphate (guanylate, guanylic acid)
GM&S	general medical and surgical
GMT	geometric mean titer
GMW	gram molecular weight
GN	glomerulonephritis • gonococcus • graduate nurse • gram-negative
G/N	glucose-nitrogen ratio
GNB	Gram negative bacillus
GNC	General Nursing Council • Gram negative cocci
gnd	ground
GND	Gram negative diplococci
GNP	gerontological nurse-practitioner
GNR	Gram negative rods
GnRH	gonadotropin-releasing hormone
GNS	gerontological nurse-specialist
GNTP	graduate nurse transition program
GO	glucose oxidase
GOE	gas, oxygen, ether
GOK	God only knows
GOR	general operating room
GOT	glutamic-oxaloacetic transaminase
govt	government
GP	general paralysis • general paresis • general practice, general practitioner • gram-positive • group • guinea pig
GPB	glossopharyngeal breathing
GPC	gastric parietal cells • Gram positive cocci
G-6-PD	glucose-6-phosphate dehydrogenase
GPEP	General Professional Education of the Physician

GPI	general paralysis of the insane • Gingival-Periodontal Index
GPM	general preventive medicine
GPN	graduate practical nurse
GPO	group purchasing organization
GPPP	group practice prepayment plan
GPR	Gram positive rods
GPT	glutamic-pyruvic transaminase
GpTh	group therapy
gr	grain • gravity
Gr	Greek
GR	gamma ray • gastric resection • general relief
GRA	Gombarts reducing agent
grad	by degrees • gradient • gradually • graduate
GRAE	generally recognized as effective
GRAN ·	Gombarts reducing agent - negative
GRAS	generally recognized as safe
grav	gravid, gravida • gravity
GRAY	Gombarts reducing agent - positive
GRE	Graduate Record Examination
GR-FeSV	Gardner-Rasheed feline sarcoma virus
GRH	growth hormone-releasing hormone
GRID	Gay-Related Immune Deficiency
GRN	geriatric resource nurse
GRS ·	gross
GRS & MIC	gross and microscopic
GRT	graduate respiratory therapist
GS	gallstone • general surgeon, general surgery • glomerular sclerosis

GSA	Gerontological Society of America
GSC	gas-solid chromatography
GSE	gluten-sensitive enteropathy • grips strong and equal
GSH	glutathione, reduced form
GSR	galvanic skin response • generalized Shwartzman reaction
GSSG	glutathione, oxidized form
GSW	gunshot wound
gt	drop (*gutta*)
GT	gait training • gastrostomy tube • glucose tolerance
GTF	glucose tolerance factor
GTH	gonadotropic hormone
GTN	glomerulotubulonephritis
GTP	guanosine triphosphate
GTR	granulocyte turnover rate
gtt	drops (*guttae*)
GTT	gelatin-tellurite-taurocholate (agar) • glucose tolerance test
GU	gastric ulcer • genitourinary • gonococcal urethritis
guid	guidance
GUS	genitourinary system
GV	gentian violet
GVA	general visceral afferent
GVE	general visceral efferent
GVH	graft-versus-host
GVHD	graft-versus-host disease
GVHR	graft-versus-host reaction
GW	gigawatt
G/W	glucose in water

GXT	graded exercise test
Gy	gray
GY	gynecological disease
Gyn	gynecologic, gynecology, gynecologist

H

h	height • high • horizontal • hour • hypermetropia • hyperopia, hyperopic • hypodermic • Planck's constant
H	height • henry (unit of electrical inductance) • heroin • histamine • history • Holzknecht unit • husband • hydrogen
^{2}**H**	deuterium
^{3}**H**	tritium
H$_1$	histamine receptor type 1
H$_2$	histamine receptor type 2
H$^+$	hydrogen ion
Ha	hahnium
HA	headache • heated aerosol • hemadsorbent • hemagglutination • hepatic adenoma • hepatitis A • hyaluronic acid • hyperalimentation
HA1	hemadsorption virus, type 1
HA2	hemadsorption virus, type 2
HAA	hepatitis A antibody • hepatitis-associated antigen
HAAb	hepatitis A antibody
HAAg	hepatitis A antigen
HABA	hydroxyazobenzenebenzoic acid
HAD	hospital administration
HAE	hereditary angioneurotic edema
HAGG	hyperimmune antivariola gamma globulin
HAI	hemagglutination inhibition
halluc	hallucination
HaMSV	Harvey murine sarcoma virus

HANE	hereditary angioneurotic edema
harm	harmonic
HAP	home antibiotic program • Hospital Accreditation Program
HARPPS	Heat, Absence of use, Redness, Pain, Pus, Swelling (symptoms of infection)
HAS	hypertensive arteriosclerosis
HASHD	hypertensive arteriosclerotic heart disease
HASP	Hospital Admission and Surveillance Program
HAT	hospital arrival time
HATG	horse anti-human thymocyte globulin
HATT	hemagglutination treponemal test
HAV	hepatitis A virus
Hb	hemoglobin
HB	heart block • hemoglobin • hepatitis B • His bundle • hospital based
H-B	Hill-Burton Act (funds)
HbA	normal adult hemoglobin
HBAb	hepatitis B antibody
HBAg	hepatitis B antigen
HbAS	hemoglobin A and hemoglobin S (sickle-cell trait)
HBcAB	antibody to hepatitis B core antigen
HbCO	carboxyhemoglobin
HBD	has·been drinking • hydroxybutyrate dehydrogenase
HBDH	hydroxybutyrate dehydrogenase
HBeAg	hepatitis B e antigen
HbF	fetal hemoglobin
HBGM	home blood glucose monitoring
HBI	hepatobiliary imaging
HBIG	hepatitis B immune globulin

HbO$_2$	oxyhemoglobin
HBO	hospital benefits organization • hyperbaric oxygen
HBP	high blood pressure • hospital based physician
HbS	sickle-cell hemoglobin • sulfhemoglobin
HBsAB	antibody to hepatitis B surface antigen
HBsAg	hepatitis B surface antigen
HBV	hepatitis B vaccine • hepatitis B virus
HC	head compression • health care • Hickman catheter • high-calorie • home care • hospital corps • hospital course • house call • hydranencephaly • hydrocodone • hydrocortisone • hypertrophic cardiomyopathy
HCA	health care assistant
HCC	health-care corporation • hepatocellular carcinoma
HCD	health care delivery • heavy-chain disease
HCEC	Hospital Care Evaluation Committee
HCFA	Health Care Financing Administration
hCG	human chorionic gonadotropin
HCG	human chorionic gonadotropin
HCHO	formaldehyde
HCl	hydrochloric acid
HCL	hairy-cell leukemia
HCM	hypertrophic cardiomyopathy
HCN	hydrocyanic acid
HCO$_3$	bicarbonate
HCP	hereditary coproporphyria • hexachlorophene
HCPCS	HCFA Common Procedures Coding System
HCPOTP	health care practitioner other than physician
HCRIS	Hospital Cost Report Information System
hCS	human chorionic somatomammotropin

HCS	human chorionic somatomammotropin
hCT	human calcitonin • human chorionic thyrotropin
Hct	hematocrit
HCT	hematocrit • human calcitonin • human chorionic thyrotropin
HCTZ	hydrochlorothiazide
HCV	Hepatitis C virus
HCVD	hypertensive cardiovascular disease
HCW	health care worker
hd	at bedtime *(hora decubitus)*
HD	Hansen's disease • hearing distance • heart disease • hemodialysis • herniated disc • high density • hip disarticulation • Hodgkin's disease
HDC	histidine decarboxylase • human diploid cell
HDCS	human diploid-cell strain
HDCV	human diploid-cell vaccine
HDF	host defensive factor
HDL	high-density lipoprotein
HDL-C	high-density lipoprotein cholesterol
HDLP	high-density lipoprotein
HDLW	distance at which a watch is heard by the left ear
HDN	hemolytic disease of the newborn
HDRW	distance at which a watch is heard by the right ear
HDS	health delivery system
HDV	hepatitis-D virus
HDU	hemodialysis unit
He	helium
HE	hemoglobin electrophoresis • hereditary elliptocytosis
H&E	hematoxylin and eosin (stain) • heredity and environment

HEAT	human erythrocyte agglutination test
HEC	hospital ethics committee
HED	unit of roentgen-ray dosage *(Haut-Einheits-Dosis)*
HEDIS	Health plan Employer Data and Information Set
HEENT	Head, Eyes, Ears, Nose and Throat
HEK	human embryonic kidney
HEL	human embryonic lung
HeLa cells	cultured strain of carcinoma cells used for study
HELLP	Hemolysis, Elevated Liver enzymes, Low Platelets syndrome
Hem	hemolysis, hemolytic • hemorrhage • hemorrhoids
hemi	hemiplegia
HEMPAS	hereditary erythroblastic multinuclearity with positive acidified serum
HEPA	high-efficiency particulate air
HES	hydroxyethyl starch • hypereosinophilic syndrome
HeSCA	Health Sciences Communications Association
HETP	hexaethyltetraphosphate
HEV	hepatitis-E virus • human enteric virus
HEW	Health, Education and Welfare
HEX	Handicapped Educational Exchange
Hf	hafnium • half
HF	Hageman factor • hard-filled (capsules) • heart failure • hemorrhagic factor • high-frequency
HFAK	hollow-fiber artificial kidney
HFC	hard-filled capsules
HFJV	high-frequency jet ventilation
HFOV	high-frequency oscillatory ventilation
HFPPV	high-frequency positive-pressure ventilation
Hfr	high frequency

HFRS	hemorrhagic fever with renal syndrome
HFUPR	hourly fetal urine production rate
HFV	high-frequency ventilation
Hg	hemoglobin • mercury
HG	human gonadotropin
Hgb	hemoglobin
HgbF	fetal hemoglobin
HGF	human growth factor • hyperglycemic-glycogenolytic factor (glucagon)
hGG	human gamma globulin
HGG	human gamma globulin
HGH	human growth hormone
HGO	hepatic glucose output
HGP	hypogastric plexus
HG-PRT	hypoxanthine-guanine phospho-ribosyl-transferase
HH	hard of hearing • home hyperalimentation
H/H	hemoglobin/hematocrit
HHA	home health agency • home health aide
HHb	reduced hemoglobin
HHC	home health care
HHD	hypertensive heart disease
HHFM	high-humidity face mask
HHN	hand-held nebulizer • home health nurse
HHNKS	hyperglycemic, hyperosmolar nonketotic syndrome
HHO	home health organization
HHS	Health and Human Services (Department) • home health services
HHT	hereditary hemorrhagic telangiectasia
HI	health insurance • hemagglutination inhibition • hepatic insufficiency

HIAA	hydroxyindoleacetic acid
5-HIAA	5-hydroxyindoleacetic acid
HIC	health information center • health insurance claims • health insurance company
H-ICD-A	Hospital (version)-International Classification of Diseases-Adapted
HICN	cyanmethemoglobin
HID	headache, insomnia, depression
HIFC	hog intrinsic factor concentrate
HiHb	hemiglobin
H inf	hypodermoclysis infusion
HIOMT	hydroxyindole-O-methyl transferase
HIP	health insurance plan
HIPP	Health Insurance Premium Program
HiPro	high-protein
His	histidine
HIS	Hospital Information Service
Hist	histidinemia • history
HIV	human immunodeficiency virus
HIVD	herniated intervertebral disc
HJ	Howell-Jolly bodies
HJR	hepatojugular reflux
HK	human kidney (cells)
H-K	hand-to-knee (coordination)
HKO	hip-knee orthosis (splint)
hl	hectoliter
HI	hypermetropia, latent • hyperopia, latent
HL	half-life • hearing level • hearing loss • hectoliter • hyperlipidemia

H/L	heparin lock • latent hyperopia • low risk heart disease
H&L	heart and lung
HLA	histocompatibility leukocyte antigen • histo-compatibility locus antigen • homologous leukocytic antibodies • human leukocyte antigen • human lymphocyte antigen
HLA-A,B, C,D	varieties of human leukocyte antigen
HLA-DR	human histocompatibility leukocyte antigen
hLH	human luteinizing hormone
HLI	hemolysis inhibition
HLP	hyperlipoproteinemia
HLR	heart-lung resuscitation
HLTK	Holmium YAG laser thermokeratoplasty
hm	hectometer
HM	severe chronic heart disease
Hm	manifest hypermetropia • manifest hyperopia
HMC	heroin, morphine, cocaine
HMD	hyaline membrane disease
HME	heat, massage, exercise
HMEIA	Health Manpower Education Initiative Award
hMG	human menopausal gonadotropin
HMG	human menopausal gonadotropin
HMG-CoA	3-hydroxy 3-methylglutaryl coenzyme-A reductase
HMI	healed myocardial infarction
HMM	hexamethylmelamine
HMO	health maintenance organization • heart minute output
HMP	hexose monophosphate
HMPG	hydroxymethoxyphenylglycol

HMSA	Health Manpower Shortage Area
HMW	high-molecular-weight
HMX	heat, massage, exercise
hn	tonight *(hoc nocte)*
HN	head nurse
H&N	head and neck
HN$_2$	mechlorethamine (nitrogen mustard)
HNP	herniated nucleus pulposus
hnRNA	heterogeneous nuclear ribonucleic acid
HNV	has not voided
Ho	holmium
HO	house officer
h/o	history of
HO-1/ HO-2	first-year house officer, second year house officer
H$_2$0	water
H$_2$0$_2$	hydrogen peroxide
HOB	head of bed
HOCM	hypertrophic obstructive cardiomyopathy
hoc vesp	tonight *(hoc vespere)*
HOD	hyperbaric oxygen drenching
Hoff	Hoffman (reflex)
HOH	hard of hearing
HOME	Home Observation for the Management of the Environment • home-oriented maternity experience
homolat	homolateral
HOP	high oxygen pressure
HOPA	hospital-based organ procurement agency
HOPD	hospital out-patient department

HOPE	healthcare options plan entitlement
hor	horizontal
hor decub	at bedtime *(hora decubitus)*
hor interm	at the intermediate hours *(horis intermediis)*
horiz	horizontal
hor som	at bedtime *(hora somni)*
hor un spatio	at the end of an hour *(horae unius spatio)*
hosp	hospital, hospitalization
HOT	human old tuberculin
hp	horsepower
Hp	haptoglobin
HP	health plan • health professional • hemiparesis • hemiplegia • highly purified • high potency • high power • high pressure • hot pack • hot pad • house physician • hydrostatic pressure • hyperphoria • hypoparathyroidism
H&P	history and physical
HPA	hypothalamic-pituitary-adrenal (axis)
HPD	hematoporphyrin derivative
H&PE	history and physical examination
hpf	high power field
HPF	high power field
HPFH	hereditary persistence of fetal hemoglobin
hPG	human pituitary gonadotropin
HPG	human pituitary gonadotropin
HPGe	high-purity germanium
HPI	history of present illness
hPL	human placental lactogen
HPL	human placental lactogen

HPLC	high-performance liquid chromatography • high-pressure liquid chromatography
HPM	Harding-Passey melanoma
hpn	hypertension
HPN	hypertension • home parenteral nutrition
HPO	high-pressure oxygen (hyperbaric oxygen)
HPP	hereditary pyropoikilocytosis
HPPH	hydroxyphenylphenylhydantoin
HPR	hospital peer review
HPRT	hypoxanthine-guanine phosphoribosyl transferase
HPS	Hanta-virus pulmonary syndrome
HPT	hyperparathyroidism
HPTH	hyperparathyroidism
HPV	human Papillomavirus
HPVD	hypertensive pulmonary vascular disease
HPX	high-peroxide-containing(cells)
hr	hour
HR	heart rate • hemorrhagic retinopathy • human resources
HRA	Health Resources Administration • high right atrial (ECG recording)
HRCT	high resolution computer tomography
HRG	Health Research Group
HRIG	human rabies immune globulin
HRL	head rotated left
HRLA	human reovirus-like agent
HRR	Hardy-Rand-Rittler (color vision test kit) • head rotated right
HRS	hepatorenal syndrome
HRSA	Health Resources and Services Administration

HRT	hormone replacement therapy
hs	at bedtime *(hora somni)* • half-strength
HS	half-strength • heart sounds • heme synthetase • hereditary spherocytosis • herpes simplex • house surgeon • severe acute heart disease
HSA	Hazardous Substances Act • Health Services Administration • health services area • human serum albumin • hypersomnia-sleep apnea (syndrome)
HSC	Hand-Schüller-Christian
HSCD	Hand-Schüller-Christian disease
HSDI	Health Self Determination Index
HSE	herpes simplex encephalitis
HSG	herpes simplex genitalis • hysterosalpingogram
HSL	herpes simplex labialis
HSM	hepatosplenomegaly • holosystolic murmur
HSN	Hanson-Street nail • herpes simplex neonatorium
HSP	Health Systems Plan • Henoch-Schönlein purpura • Hospital Specific Payment
HSQ	home screening questionnaire
HSQB	Health Standards and Quality Bureau
HSR	homogeneously staining regions
HSS	Hallervorden-Spatz syndrome
HSTS	human-specific thyroid stimulator
HSV	herpes simplex virus • highly selective vagotomy
ht	height
Ht	hypermetropia, total • hyperopia, total
HT	Hashimoto's thyroiditis • histologic technician • home treatment • Hubbard tank • hydrotherapy • hydroxytryptamine • hypertropia • hypodermic tablet
5-HT	5-hydroxytryptamine

HTB	hot tub bath
HTL	histologic technologist
HTLV	human T-cell leukemia virus • human T-cell lymphotropic virus
HTN	hypertension
HTP	House-Tree-Person (test) • hydroxytryptophan
hTS	human thyroid stimulator
HTS	hemangioma-thrombocytopenia syndrome
HU	heat unit • hydroxyurea • hyperemia unit
HuIFN	human interferon
HUIS	high-dose urea in invert sugar
HUM	heat, ultrasound, massage
HUP	Hospital Utilization Project
HURT	hospital utilization review team
HUS	hemolytic-uremic syndrome
HV	Hanta virus • high-voltage • hospital visit • hyperventilation
HVA	homovanillic acid
HVD	hypertensive vascular disease
HVE	hepatic vascular exclusion • high-voltage electrophoresis
HVH	herpesvirus hominis
HVHMA	herpesvirus hominis membrane antigen
HVL	half-value layer
HVT	half-value thickness
HWB	hot water bottle
HWS	hot-water soluble
Hx	history • hypoxanthine
HXM	hexamethylmelamine
hy	hysteria

Hy	hydraulics • hydrostatics • hypermetropia • hyperopia
hyd	hydration
hydro	hydrotherapy
hyg	hygiene
hyp	hydroxyproline • hyperresonance • hypertrophy,
hyperten	hypertension
hypn	hypertension
hypno	hypnosis
hypo	hypodermic injection
hys	hysteria, hysterical
hyst	hysterectomy
Hz	hertz
HZ	herpes zoster
HZFO	hamster zona-free ovum (test)
HZV	herpes zoster virus

I

i	incisor (deciduous)
I	inactive • incisor (permanent) • increased • index • induction • insoluble • inspiration, inspired (gas) • intake • intensity (electrical, luminous, magnetic, radioactive) • internal medicine • internist • iodine
I$_2$	iodine
^{125}I, ^{131}I	radioactive isotopes of iodine commonly used in medicine
^{127}I	stable iodine
IA	immunobiologic activity • impedance angle • incurred accidentally • infantile apnea • intra-amniotic • intra-aortic • intra-arterial • intra-articular
IAA	indoleacetic acid
IABC	intra-aortic balloon counterpulsation
IABP	intra-aortic balloon pump
IABPA	intra-aortic balloon-pumping assistance
I-Ac	imideazoleacetic acid
IAC	internal auditory canal • interposed abdominal compression
IADH	inappropriate antidiuretic hormone
IADL	Instrumental Activities of Daily Living (scale)
IAEA	International Atomic Energy Agency
IAET	International Association for Enterostomal Therapy
IAFI	infantile amaurotic familial idiocy
IAHA	immune-adherence hemagglutination
i-amniot	intra-amniotic

IANC	International Anatomical Nomenclature Committee
IAP	intermittent acute porphyria
IARC	International Agency for Research on Cancer
i-arter	intra-arterial
IAS	intra-amniotic saline (infusion)
IASD	interatrial septal defect
IAT	indirect antiglobulin test • iodine-azide test
IAV	intermittent assisted ventilation
IB	immune body • inclusion body • index of body build • infectious bronchitis
IBC	iron-binding capacity
IBD	infectious bowel disease • inflammatory bowel disease
IBF	immunoglobulin-binding factor
IBI	intermittent bladder irrigation
ibid	the same, in the same place *(ibidem)*
IBNR	incurred but not reported
IBP	iron-binding protein
IBR	infectious bovine rhinotracheitis
IBS	irritable bowel syndrome
IBU	international benzoate unit
IBV	infectious bronchitis virus
IBW	ideal body weight
ic	between meals *(inter cibos)*
IC	infection control • information content • inhibitory concentration • inspiratory capacity • inspiratory center • intensive care • intercarpal • intercostal • intermediate care • interstitial cell • intracarotid • intracellular • intracerebral • intracranial • intracutaneous • intraductal carcinoma • irritable colon
IC$_{50}$	median inhibitory concentration

iCA	ionized calcium
ICA	intercountry adoption • internal carotid artery
i-card	intracardial
ICC	intensive coronary care • intermittent clean catheterization
ICCE	intracapsular cataract extraction
ICCU	intensive coronary care unit
ICD	implantable cardioverter defibrillator • International Classification of Diseases • isocitric dehydrogenase
ICD-A	International Classification of Diseases - Adapted
ICD-9	International Classification of Diseases - Ninth Revision
ICD-9-CM	International Classification of Diseases - Ninth Revision - Clinical Modification
ICDH	isocitric dehydrogenase
ICE	ifosfamide, carboplatin, etoposide
ICES	ice, compression, elevation, support
ICF	intermediate-care facility • intracellular fluid
ICF/MR	intermediate-care facility for the mentally retarded
ICG	indocyanine green
ICM	intercostal margin
ICN	intensive care nursery • International Council of Nurses
i-coch	intracochlear
ICP	infection control practitioner • intracranial pressure
ICPMM	incisors, canines, premolars, molars
ICR	distance between iliac crests • intrastromal corneal ring
ICRC	infant care review committee
ICRP	International Commission on Radiological Protection

ICRU	International Commission on Radiological Units and Measurements
ICS	intercostal space • International College of Surgeons
ICSH	interstitial cell-stimulating hormone (luteinizing hormone)
ict	icterus
iCT	immunoreactive calcitonin
ICT	inflammation of connective tissue • insulin-coma therapy • intensive conventional therapy
ict ind	icterus index
ICU	infant care unit • intermediate care unit • intensive care unit
i-cut	intracutaneous
ICW	intensive care ward • intracellular water
id	the same (*idem*)
ID	identification • immunodiffusion • immunoglobulin deficiency • inclusion disease • infectious disease • infective dose • inhibitory dose • inside diameter • intradermal
I&D	incision and drainage
ID$_{50}$	median infective dose
IDA	iminodiacetic acid • iron-deficiency anemia
IDAT	indirect antiglobulin test
IDD	insulin-dependent diabetes
IDDF	investigational drug data form
IDDM	insulin-dependent diabetes mellitus
IDDS	investigational drug data sheet
IDE	investigational drug exemption
i-derm	intradermal
IDL	intermediate-density lipoproteins
IDM	infant of diabetic mother

IDP	inosine diphosphate
IDT	intradermal test
IDU	idoxuridine
IDUR	idoxuridine
IDV	intermittent demand ventilation
ie	that is *(id est)*
IE	immunoelectrophoresis • infective endocarditis
I/E	inspiratory/expiratory
IEA	intravascular erythrocyte aggregation
IEC	intra-epithelial carcinoma
IED	intermittent explosive disorder
IEE	inner enamel epithelium
IEF	isoelectric focusing
IEM	inborn error of metabolism
IEOP	immunoelectro-osmophoresis
IEP	immunoelectrophoresis • isoelectric point
IF	immunofluorescence • inhibiting factor • initiation factor • interferon • intermediate frequency • interstitial fluid • intrinsic factor • involved-field (radiotherapy)
IFA	immunofluorescent assay • indirect fluorescent antibody
IFE	immunofixation electrophoresis
IFN	interferon
iG	immunoreactive gastrin
Ig	immunoglobulin
IG	immune globulin • immunoglobulin • Inspector General
IgA	immunoglobulin A
IgD	immunoglobulin D
IgE	immunoglobulin E

IGF	insulin-like growth factor
IGFBP	IGF-binding proteins
IgG	immunoglobulin G
IGIV	immune globulin intravenous
IgM	immunoglobulin M
IgQ	immunoglobulin quantitation
IGR	intrauterine growth retardation
IGT	impaired glucose tolerance
IH	indirect hemagglutination • infectious hepatitis • inhibiting hormone • inpatient hospital
IHA	immune hemolytic anemia • indirect hemagglutination
IHD	ischemic heart disease
IHO	idiopathic hypertrophic osteoarthropathy • Institute of Human Origins
IHP	idiopathic hypopituitarism
IHSA	iodinated human serum albumin
^{131}**IHSA**	radioiodinated (radioactive iodine-labeled) human serum albumin
IHSS	idiopathic hypertrophic subaortic stenosis • In-Home Support Services
II	icterus indes • image intensifier • insurance index
IICP	increased intracranial pressure
IICU	infant intensive care unit
IID	insulin-independent diabetes
IIE	idiopathic ineffective erythropoiesis
IIF	indirect immunofluorescence
IIIVC	infrahepatic interruption of the inferior vena cava
IIS	intermittent infusion sets
I-J	ileojejunal

IL	incisolingual • independent laboratory • insensible weight loss • interleukin • intermediary letter
ILA	insulin-like activity
I-Lac	imidazolelactic acid
ILBBB	incomplete left bundle branch block
IIc	isoleucine
i-lesion	intralesional
IM	Index Medicus • infectious mononucleosis • internal medicine • intramedullary • intramuscular
IMA	Industrial Medicine Association
IMC	immediate care
IMCU	intermediate care unit
ImD$_{50}$	median immunizing dose
IME	indirect medical education
IMF	intermaxillary fixation
IMI	immunologically measurable insulin
immat	immature
immed	immediate
immob	immobilize
ImmU	immunizing unit
immunol	immunology, immunological
IMN	internal mammary nodes
imp	important • impression • improved
IMP	incomplete male pseudohermaphroditism • inosine monophosphate
IMPA	incisal mandibular plane angle
impair	impaired, impairment
Impx.	impaction
IMR	infectious mononucleosis receptors

IMS	Indian Medical Services
IMSC	internal mammary supraclavicular
ImU	international milliunit
IMV	intermittent mandatory ventilation
IMViC	indole, methyl red, Voges-Proskauer, citrate
in	inch
In	indium
IN	icterus neonatorum • internist • intranasal
INAH	isoniazid (isonicotinic acid hydrazide)
inc	incomplete • inconclusive • incontinent • increase
Inc AB	incomplete abortion
incl	including • inclusive
IncO$_2$	incubator oxygen
incompat	incompatible
incompl	incomplete
incr	increase, increased, increasing • increment
inc(R)	increase (relative)
incur	incurable
in d	daily *(in dies)*
ind	independent
IND	Investigational New Drug
indic	indicative, indication
INDM	infant of nondiabetic mother
indust	industry, industrial
inf	infant, infancy, infantile • infect, infected, infection, infectious • inferior • infirmary • infusion • pour in *(infunde)*
infarct	infarction
inf dis	infectious disease

infect	infection, infectious
infl	influence
inflam	inflamed, inflammation, inflammatory
info	information
infx	infection
ing	inguinal
ingest	ingestion
inh	inhalation
INH	isoniazid (isonicotinic acid hydrazide)
inhal	inhalation
inhib	inhibit, inhibition, inhibitor
INI	intranasal insulin • intranuclear inclusion (agent)
inj	inject, injection • injury, injurious
inject	injection
inj enem	let an enema be given *(injiciatur enema)*
in-lb	inch-pound
INN	International Nonproprietary Names
innerv	innervation, innerved
Ino	inosine
inoc	inoculate, inoculated, inoculation
inop	inoperable
inorg	inorganic
Inorg phos	inorganic phosphorus
INPRONS	information processing in the central nervous system
INR	International Normalized Ratio
INS	insert • insurance
insol	insoluble
insp	inspiration
inst	institute • instrument

instil	instilled, instillation
instr	instructor
insuff	insufficiency, insufficient
int	integral • intermittent • internal • internist • intestinal
int cib	between meals *(inter cibos)*
intest	intestine, intestinal
Int FHR	internal fetal heart rate
INTH	intrathecal
Int Med	internal medicine
intox	intoxication
int rot	internal rotation
in utero	within the uterus
inv	inverse • inversion • involuntary
Io	ionium
IO	inferior oblique • intestinal obstruction • intraocular
I&O	intake and output
IOC	intern on call
IOFB	intraocular foreign body
IOL	intraocular lens
IOML	infraorbitomeatal line
IOP	intraocular pressure
IOPA	independent organ procurement agency
IORT	intraoperative radiotherapy
IOTA	information overload testing aid
IOV	initial office visit
IP	incisoproximal • incubation period • infection prevention • initial pressure • inpatient • International Pharmacopeia • interphalangeal • intraperitoneal • isoelectric point

IPA	independent practice association • individual practice association • isopropyl alcohol
IPD	immediate pigment darkening • intermittent peritoneal dialysis
IPE	interstitial pulmonary emphysema
i-periton	intraperitoneal
IPF	infection-potentiating factor
IPG	impedance plethysmography
IPH	idiopathic pulmonary hemosiderosis • interphalangeal
IPJ	interphalangeal joint
IPL	interpupillary line
i-pleur	intrapleural
IPN	interim progress note
IPP	inpatient pharmacy • intermittent positive pressure
IPPA	inspection, palpation, percussion, auscultation
IPPB	intermittent positive-pressure breathing
IPPBA	intermittent positive-pressure breathing apparatus
IPPF	International Planned Parenthood Foundation
IPPR	intermittent positive-pressure respiration
IPPV	intermittent positive-pressure ventilation
IPR	independent professional review
IPRA	Independent Professional Review Agents
IPSP	inhibitory postsynaptic potential
IPTG	isopropylthiogalactoside
IPTH	immunoreactive parathyroid hormone
IPV	inactivated poliovirus vaccine
IQ	intelligence quotient
Ir	immune response (genes) • iridium

IR	immunoreactive • inferior rectus • infrared • internal resistance • internal rotation • inversion-recovery • irritant reaction
IRB	Institutional Review Board • intern/resident to bed ratio
IRBBB	incomplete right bundle branch block
IRC	inspiratory reserve capacity • International Red Cross
IRDS	idiopathic respiratory distress syndrome • infant respiratory distress syndrome
IRGI	immunoreactive glucagon
IRHGH	immunoreactive human growth hormone
IRI	immunoreactive insulin
irid	iridescent
IRI/G	ratio of immunoreactive insulin to glucose
IRM	innate releasing mechanism • Institute of Rehabilitation Medicine
IRMA	immunoradiometric assay
IRO	International Refugee Organization
IRP	immunoreactive proinsulin • Inter- national Reference Preparation
IRR	intrarenal reflux
irrig	irrigated, irrigation
IRV	inspiratory reserve volume
IS	immune serum • incentive spiro- meter • induced sputum • intensity of services • intercostal space • interspace • interventri- cular septum • intraspinal • inventory of systems • island
ISA	International Symbol of Access
ISC	International Statistical Classification • interstitial cell • irreversibly sickled cell
ISD	initial sleep disturbance • isosorbide dinitrate
ISDN	isosorbide dinitrate

ISE	ion-selective electrode
ISF	interstitial fluid
ISG	immune serum globulin
ISO	International Standards Organization
isoenz	isoenzymes
isol	isolation
isom	isometric
ISP	distance between iliac spines • intraspinal
ISR	Institute of Surgical Research
IST	insulin shock therapy
ISW	interstitial water
ISY	intrasynovial
IT	information technologies • inhalation therapy • intertrochanteric • intertuberous • intimal thickening • intrathecal • intrathoracic
ITFF	intertrochanteric femoral fracture
ITFS	incomplete testicular feminization syndrome
IT Fx	intertrochanteric fracture
i-thec	intrathecal
ITP	idiopathic thrombocytopenic purpura • inosine triphosphate
ITPA	Illinois Test of Psycholinguistic Abilities
ITQ	Infant Temperament Questionnaire
ITR	intratracheal
i-trach	intratracheal
ITT	insulin tolerance test • iron tolerance test
i-tumor	intratumoral
ITX	intertriginous xanthoma
IU	immunizing unit • international unit • intrauterine
IUCD	intrauterine contraceptive device

IUD	intrauterine death • intrauterine device
IUDR	idoxuridine
IUFB	intrauterine foreign body
IUFD	intrauterine fetal distress
IUGR	intrauterine growth rate • intrauterine growth retardation
IUP	intrauterine pregnancy
IUPAC	International Union of Pure and Applied Chemistry
IUPC	intrauterine pressure catheter
IV	interventricular • intervertebral • intravascular • intravenous • intraventricular
IVAC	intravenous automated controller
IVC	inferior vena cava • inspired vital capacity • intravenous cholangiogram, intravenous cholangiography
IVCD	intraventricular conduction defect • intraventricular conduction delay
IVD	intervertebral disk
IVF	intravascular fluid • intravenous fluid
IVGTT	intravenous glucose tolerance test
IVH	intravenous hyperalimentation
IVIG	intravenous immunoglobulin
IVJC	intervertebral joint complex
IVLBW	infant of very low birth weight
IVOX	intravascular oxygenator
IVP	intravenous pyelogram • intraventricular pressure • intravenous push
IVPB	intravenous piggyback
IVPF	isovolume pressure flow (curve)
IVS	interventricular septum
IVSD	interventricular septal defect

IVSS	intravenous Solu-Set
IVT	intravenous transfusion • isovolumic time
IVU	intravenous urography
IWI	inferior wall infarction
IWL	insensible water loss
IWMI	inferior wall myocardial infarction
IZS	insulin zinc suspension

J

J	joint • joule • Joule's equivalent • journal • juice
JAI	juvenile amaurotic idiocy
JAMA	Journal of the American Medical Association
JAN	Job Accommodation Network
jaund	jaundice
JCAH	Joint Commission on Accreditation of Hospitals
JCAHO	Joint Commission on Accreditation of Healthcare Organizations
jct	junction
JEE	Japanese equine encephalitis
jej.	jejunum
JFS	Jewish Family Services
JG	juxtaglomerular
JGA	juxtaglomerular apparatus
JI	jejunoileal
JJ	jaw jerk
JMD	juvenile macular degeneration
JND	just noticeable difference
jnt	joint
JOB	Job Opportunities for the Blind
JOC	joint operating committees
JODM	juvenile-onset diabetes mellitus
jour	journal
J-P	Jackson-Pratt drain
JPC	junctional premature contracture

JRA	juvenile rheumatoid arthritis
jt	joint
JUA	Joint Underwriting Association
junct	junction
juv	juvenile
JVD	jugular venous distention

K

k	rate or velocity constant
K	absolute zero (Kelvin) • cathode • dissociation constant • electrostatic capacity • equilibrium constant • Kelvin • keratometer • kilo- • permeability coefficient • potassium *(kalium)* • thousand (kilo)
°K	degrees Kelvin (absolute temperature)
K⁺	potassium ion
Ka	cathode • kallikrein
KA	ketoacidosis • King-Armstrong (unit)
KAFO	knee-ankle-foot orthosis
KAP	knowledge, aptitude, practices
kb	kilobase
KB	ketone bodies
K-B	Kleihauer-Betke (stain)
KBr	potassium bromide
kc	kilocycle
KC	kathodal closure • keratoconjunctivitis • kilocycle
K-C	knee-chest
kcal	kilocalorie (large calorie)
KCC	kathodal closure contraction
KCF	key clinical findings
kCi	kilocurie
KCl	potassium chloride
kcps	kilocycles per second
KCS	keratoconjunctivitis sicca

kc/sec	kilocycles per second
KCT	kathodal closure tetanus
KD	kathodal duration • knitted Dacron
K$_D$	dissociation constant
K/D	Keto-Diastix
kdal	kilodalton
KDC	Kidney Disease Treatment Center
KDT	kathodal duration tetanus
KDTC	Kidney Disease Treatment Center
KE	kinetic energy
KED	Kendrick Extrication Device
kev	kiloelectron-volt
keV	kiloelectron-volt
KFD	kinetic family drawings
kg	kilogram
kg-cal	kilogram-calorie (large calorie)
kg-m	kilogram-meter
KGS	ketogenic steroid
KHb	potassium hemoglobinate
KHN	Knoop hardness number
kHz	kilohertz
K$_i$	inhibition constant
KI	Krönig's isthmus • potassium iodide
kilo	kilogram
KiMSV	Kirsten murine sarcoma virus
kJ	kilojoule
KJ	knee jerk
KK	knee kick
kl	kiloliter

KL bac	Klebs-Löffler bacillus
KLH	keyhole-limpet hemocyanin
KLS	kidney, liver, spleen
km	kilometer
K$_m$	Michaelis constant
KM	kanamycin • Kussmaul (respirations)
kMc	kilomegacycle
kMcps	kilomegacycles per second
KMIS	keratomileusis-in-situ
KMnO$_4$	potassium permanganate
KO	keep open • knock out
KOC	kathodal opening contraction
KOH	potassium hydroxide
KP	keratitic precipitates • keratitis punctata
kPa	kilopascal (unit of pressure)
KPE	Kilman phacoemulsification
Kr	kiloroentgen • krypton
KRP	Kolmer test with Reiter protein
KS	Kaposi's sarcoma • ketosteroid • Kochleffel syndrome • kyphoscoliosis
KTP	potassium titanyl phosphate
KU	Kimbel unit
KUB	kidneys, ureters, bladder
kv	kilovolt
kV	kilovolt
kVA	kilovolt-ampere
KVO	keep vein open
kvp	kilovolts peak
kw	kilowatt

kW	kilowatt
KW	Keith-Wagener scale of retinopathy • Kirschner wire
kw-hr	kilowatt-hour
K-wire	Kirschner wire

L

l	levo- (left, counterclockwise) • liter
L	coefficient of induction • *Lactobacillus* • lateral • lambert (unit of brightness) • Latin • left (counterclockwise) • length • lethal • levorotatory • Lewisite • licensed • ligament • light • light sense • liter • low, lower, lowest • lumbar • lumen • pound *(libra)*
L1-L5	lumbar vertebrae 1 through 5
La	lanthanum
LA	lactic acid • Latin American • left angle • left arm • left atrial (pressure) • left atrium • left auricle • leucine aminopeptidase • linoleic acid • local anesthesia • long-acting
L&A	light and accommodation
LAA	left atrial abnormality • leukocyte ascorbic acid
lab	laboratory
lab proc	laboratory procedure
lac	laceration
LAC	long arm cast
lact	lactate, lactating
LAD	lactic acid dehydrogenase • left anterior descending • left axis deviation • linoleic acid depression
LADCA	left anterior descending coronary artery
LAE	left atrial enlargement
LAF	laminar air flow
LAFB	left anterior fascicular block
LAH	left anterior hemiblock • left atrial hypertrophy
LAHB	left anterior hemiblock

LAI	left atrial involvement
LAIT	latex agglutination inhibition test
LAK	lymphokine-activated killer cells
LaL	labiolingual
Lam	laminectomy
L Ant	left anterior
LAO	left anterior oblique
lap	laparotomy
LAP	left atrial pressure • leucine aminopeptidase • leukocyte alkaline phosphatase • lyophilized anterior pituitary
LAPMS	long arm posterior molded splint
LAR	left arm recumbent
LARC	leukocyte automatic recognition computer
LAS	linear alkylate sulfonate
LASER	light amplification by stimulated emission of radiation
L-Asp	L-asparaginase
LASS	labile aggregation-stimulating substance
LAST	Leukocyte-Antigen Sensitivity Testing
lat	lateral • latitude
lat dol	to the painful side (*lateri dolenti*)
LATS	long-acting thyroid stimulator
LATSP	long-acting thyroid stimulator protector
LAV	lymphadenopathy-associated virus
LAVH	laparoscopy-assisted vaginal hysterectomy
lb	pound (*libra*)
LB	laser bullectomy • live birth • low back
L-B	Liebermann-Burchard (reaction)
L&B	left and below

LBB	left breast biopsy • left bundle branch
LBBB	left bundle branch block
LBBsB	left bundle branch system block
LBBX	left breast biopsy examination
LBCD	left border of cardiac dullness
LBD	left border dullness
lb-ft	pound-feet, pound-foot
LBH	length, breadth, height
LBM	last bowel movement • lean body mass
LBNP	lower-body negative pressure
LBP	low back pain • low blood pressure
LBRF	louse-borne relapsing fever
LBT	lupus band test
LBVP	luminal balloon valvuloplasty
LBW	low birth weight
LC	laparoscopic cholecystectomy • lactation consultant • left ear, cold stimulus • leisure counseling • lethal concentration • linguocervical • liquid capsule • living children • low-calorie
LCA	left coronary artery
LCAH	life care at home
LCAT	lecithin-cholesterol-acyltransferase (deficiency)
LCCA	left common carotid artery
LCCS	low cervical cesarean section
LCD	liquid-crystal display
LCFA	long-chain fatty acid
LCGME	Liaison Committee on Graduate Medical Education
LCh	Licentiate in Surgery (*Chirurgia*)
LCIS	lobular carcinoma in situ
LCL	Levinthal-Coles-Lille (bodies)

LCM	left costal margin • lymphocytic choriomeningitis
LCME	Liaison Committee on Medical Education
LCP	Legg-Calve-Perthes' disease
LCSW	licensed clinical social worker
LCT	lymphocytotoxicity test
LD	lactic dehydrogenase • learning disability • left deltoid • lethal dose • light difference (perception) • linguodistal • living donor • low dosage • Lyme disease
LD$_{50}$	median lethal dose
LDA	left dorsoanterior
LDB	legionnaires' disease bacterium
LDC	leukocyte differential count
LDH	lactic dehydrogenase
LDL	low-density lipoprotein
LDL-C	low-density lipoprotein cholesterol
LDLP	low-density lipoprotein
LDP	left dorsoposterior
LDR	labor, delivery, recovery
LDRP	labor, delivery, recovery, post-partum
LDS	Licentiate in Dental Surgery
Le	Leonard (cathode ray unit)
LE	left eye • lower extremity • lupus erythematosus
LED	light-emitting diode • lupus erythematosus disseminatus
LES	local excitatory state • lower esophageal sphincter
LET	linear energy transfer
Leu	leucine
lev	levator muscle
Lf	limit of flocculation (unit)

LF	low forceps (delivery) • low frequency
LFA	left femoral artery • left forearm • left frontoanterior
LFD	least fatal dose • low fat diet • low forceps delivery
LFH	left femoral hernia
LFL	left frontolateral
LFP	left frontoposterior
LFPS	Licentiate of the Faculty of Physicians and Surgeons
LFT	latex flocculation test • left frontotransverse • liver function test
lg	large
LG	laryngectomy • left gluteal, left gluteus • linguogingival
LGA	large for gestational age
LGB	Landry-Guillain-Barré (syndrome)
LGH	lactogenic hormone
LGL	Lown-Ganong-Levine (syndrome)
LGN	lateral geniculate nucleus
LGV	lymphogranuloma venereum
LH	left hand • luteinizing hormone • lues hereditaria
LHH	left homonymous hemianopsia
LHP	left hemiparesis • left hemiplegia
LHRF	luteinizing hormone-releasing factor
LHRH	luteinizing hormone-releasing hormone
LHS	left heart strain
LHV	left hepatic vein
Li	lithium
LIA	leukemia-associated inhibitory activity • lysine-iron agar
LIBC	latent iron-binding capacity

LIC	left iliac crest • left internal carotid • leisure-interest class
LICA	left internal carotid artery
LICM	left intercostal margin
LICS	left intercostal space
LIF	left iliac fossa • leukocyte inhibitory factor
LIFE	Longitudinal Interval Follow-up Evaluation
lig	ligament
LIH	left inguinal hernia
LIMA	left internal mammary artery
lin	linear
linim	liniment
LIP	lymphoid interstitial pneumonia
liq	liquid • liquor
LIRBM	liver, iron, red bone marrow
LIS	lobular in situ • low intermittent suction
LISS	low-ionic-strength saline solution
lith	lithotomy
LK	lamellar keratectomy • left kidney
LKS	liver, kidneys, spleen
LL	left lateral • left leg • left lung • lepromatous leprosy • lower lid
LLat	left lateral
L LAT	left lateral
LLB	long-leg brace
LLBCD	left lower border of cardiac dullness
LLC	long-leg cast • lower level of care
LLD	*Lactobacillus lactis*, Dorner factor (vitamin B12) • left lateral decubitus (position)
LLE	left lower extremity

LLL	left lower lobe
LLLI	La Leche League International
LLM	localized leukocyte mobilization
LLO	*Legionella*-like organisms
LLPMS	long leg posterior molded splint
LLQ	left lower quadrant
LLR	left lateral rectus
LLSB	left lower sternal border
LLT	left lateral thigh
lm	lumen
LM	Licentiate in Midwifery • light microscopy • linguomesial • longitudinal muscle
LMA	left mentoanterior
LMB	Laurence-Moon-Biedl syndrome • left mainstem bronchus
LMC	lymphocyte-mediated cytotoxicity
LMCA	left main coronary artery
LMCL	left midclavicular line
LMD	local medical doctor
LMF	lymphocytic mitogenic factor
LMHT	licensed mental health technician
LMI	leukocyte migration inhibition
LML	left mediolateral
LMM	lentigo maligna melanoma
LMP	last menstrual period • left mentoposterior
LMS	Licentiate in Medicine and Surgery
LMT	left mentotransverse • leukocyte migration technique
lmtd	limited
LMW	low molecular weight

LMWD	low molecular weight dextran
LN	lobular neoplasia • lymph node
LNC	lymph-node cells
LNMP	last normal menstrual period
LNPF	lymph node permeability factor
LO	linguo-occlusal
LOA	leave of absence • left occipitoanterior
LOC	laxative of choice • level of consciousness • loss of consciousness
loc cit	in the place cited *(loco citato)*
loc dol	to the painful spot *(loco dolenti)*
LoCHO	low carbohydrate
LoChol	low cholesterol
LOD	line of duty
log	logarithm
LOH	length of hospitalization
LOM	limitation of motion • loss of motion
LOMSA	left otitis media suppurative, acute
LOMSCh	left otitis media suppurative, chronic
LoNa⁺	low sodium
long	longitudinal
LOP	leave on pass • left occipitoposterior
LOQ	lower outer quadrant
LOR	loss of resistance
LOS	length of stay
lot	lotion
LOT	left occipitotransverse

LP	latent period • leukocytic pyrogen • light perception • lipoprotein • low power • low pressure • lumbar puncture • lymphoid predominance
L/P	lactate-pyruvate ratio
LPA	left pulmonary artery
L-PAM	L-phenylalanine mustard
lpf	low-power field
LPF	leukocytosis-promoting factor • low-power field
LPFB	left posterior fascicular block
LPH	left posterior hemiblock
LPHB	left posterior hemiblock
lpi	lines per inch
LPICA	left posterior internal carotid artery
lpm	lines per minute • liters per minute
LPM	liters per minute
LPN	licensed practical nurse
LPO	left posterior oblique
L POST	left posterior
LPS	Lanterman-Petris-Short • levator palpebrae superioris (muscle) • lipase • lipopolysaccharide
LPV	left portal vein
LQ	left quadrant
Lr	lawrencium
LR	lactated Ringer's • latency relaxation • lateral rectus (muscle)
L-R	left to right
L/R	left/right
LRC	Lipid Research Center
LRCP	Licentiate of the Royal College of Physicians
LRCS	Licentiate of the Royal College of Surgeons

LRD	living related donor
LRE	leukemic reticuloendotheliosis
LRF	liver residue factor • luteinizing hormone-releasing factor
LRH	luteinizing hormone-releasing hormone
LRI	lower respiratory infection
LRQ	lower right quadrant
LRR	labyrinthine righting reflex
LS	lumbosacral
L/S	lecithin-sphingomyelin ratio • liver-spleen
LSA	left sacroanterior • left subclavian artery • Licentiate of the Society of Apothecaries
LSB	left sternal border
LScA	left scapuloanterior
LScP	left scapuloposterior
LSD	least significant digit • lysergic acid diethylamide
LSH	luetin-stimulating hormone • lymphocyte-stimulating hormone
LSK	liver, spleen, kidneys
LSM	lysergic acid morpholide
LSO	left salpingo-oophorectomy • lumbosacral orthosis
LSP	left sacroposterior
LSS	liver-spleen scan • lumbosacral spine
LST	lateral sinus thrombophlebitis • left sacrotransverse
LSU	life-support unit
LSW	left-sided weakness
lt	left • light • low tension
LT	left triceps • leukotriene • locum tenens • lymphocyte transformation • lymphocytic thyroiditis • lymphotoxin
LTA	laryngotracheal anesthesia

LTB	laryngotracheobronchitis
LTC	long-term care
LTCF	long-term care facility
LTCS	low transverse Cesarean section
LTCU	long-term care unit
LTD	limited
LTF	lipotropic factor • lymphocyte transforming factor
LTH	luteotropic hormone
LTM	long-term memory
LTP	L-tryptophan
LTPP	lipothiamide pyrophosphate
LTR	long-terminal repeat
LTT	leucine tolerance test • lymphocyte transformation test
Lu	lutetium
LU	left upper
LUCs	large unstained cells
LUE	left upper extremity
LUIS	low-dose urea in invert sugar
LUL	left upper lobe
LUO	left ureteral orifice
LUOQ	left upper outer quadrant
LUQ	left upper quadrant
LV	left ventricle, left ventricular • live vaccine
LVD	left ventricular dimension
LVE	left ventricular enlargement
LVEDP	left ventricular end-diastolic pressure
LVEDV	left ventricular end-diastolic volume
LVEF	left ventricular ejection fraction

LVET	left ventricular ejection time
LVFP	left ventricular filling pressure
LVH	large-vessel hematocrit • left ventricular hypertrophy
LVID	left ventricular internal dimension
LVIDP	left ventricular initial diastolic pressure
LVLG	left ventrolateral gluteal
LVN	licensed visiting nurse • licensed vocational nurse
LVO	left ventricular outflow • left ventricular overactivity
LVP	left ventricular pressure
LVSW	left ventricular stroke work
LVSWI	left ventricular stroke work index
LW	left ear, warm stimulus
L&W	Lee and White (clotting time) • living and well
LWCT	Lee-White clotting time
lx	lux (illuminance unit)
Lx	local irradiation
lym	lymphocyte
Lys	lysine
lytes	electrolytes
LZM	lysozyme

M

m	handful *(manipulus)* • mass • meter • milli- • minim • minute • molar • morphine • mucoid • murmur • noon *(meridies)*
M	chin *(mentum)* • macerate(d) • male • malignant • married • massage • mature • mean • median • medical • medium • mega- • melts at • membrane • memory • metabolite • meter • method • *Micrococcus* • minim • mitral • mix, mixture • molar • molecular weight • Monday • morgan (unit of chromosome map distance) • morphine • mother • muscle • myeloma • myopia, myopic • noon *(meridies)* • thousand *(mille)*
mμ	millimicro- • millimicron
m²	square meter
m³	cubic meter
ma	milliampere
mA	milliampere
MA	mandelic acid • manifest achievement • Master of Arts • medical abbreviation • medical assistant • medical audit • membrane antigen • menstrual age • mental age • meter angle • Miller-Abbott (tube) • milliampere
MAA	macroaggregated albumin
MAB	management of assaultive behavior • monoclonal antibody
MABP	mean arterial blood pressure
mac	macerate

MAC	malignancy associated changes • maximum (maximal) allowable concentration • maximum allowable cost • methotrexate, actinomycin D, cyclo- phosphamide • mid-arm circumference • minimum alveolar concentration • minimum anesthetic concen- tration • mitral anular calcium • monitored anesthesia care • Mycobacterium avium complex
MACC	methotrexate, doxorubicin, cyclophosphamide, lomustine
MADC	mean average daily census
MADRS	Medicare automated data retrieval system
MAE	moves all extremities
MAEW	moves all extremities well
MAF	macrophage activating factor • minimum (minimal) audible field
mag	large *(magnus)* • magnification
Mag	magnesium
MAG	myelin-associated glycoprotein
MAHA	microangiopathic hemolytic anemia
MAI	*Mycobacterium avium* infection • *Mycobacterium avium intracellulare*
MAIC	*Mycobacterium avium intracellulare* complex
mall	malleolus
mam	milliampere-minute
M+Am	compound myopic astigmatism
MAMC	mid-arm muscle circumference
man	handful *(manipulus)*
mand	mandible, mandibular
manif	manifest, manifested
manip	handful *(manipulus)* • manipulation
man pr	early in the morning *(mane primo)*

MAO	maximal acid output • monoamine oxidase
MAODP	Medic Alert Organ Donor Program
MAOI	monoamine oxidase inhibitor
MAP	mean aortic pressure • mean arterial pressure • medical assistance program • medical audit program • minimum (minimal) audible pressure • monophasic action potential • muscle action potential
MAPS	Make-a-Picture Story (test)
MAR	Medication Administration Record • minimal angle resolution
MARC	Medical Air Rescue Corps
MARS	Mevinolin Atherosclerosis Regression Study
mas	milliampere-second
MaS	milliampere-second
masc	masculine
MASER	microwave amplification by stimulated emission of radiation
MASH	mobile army surgical hospital • mutual aid and self-help
mass	massage
mast	mastectomy
mAST	mitochondrial aspartate aminotransferase
MAST	Medical Anti-Shock Trousers • Michigan Alcoholism Screening Test • Military Anti-Shock Trousers
Mat	maternity
MAT	manual arts therapy, therapist • motivation analysis test
matut	in the morning *(matutimus)*
max	maxilla, maxillary • maximal, maximum
mb	mix well *(misce bene)*

Mb	myoglobin
MB	Bachelor of Medicine *(Medicinae Baccalaureus)* • Marsh-Bendall factor • methylene blue
MBA	Master of Business Administration
M-BACOD	methotrexate, bleomycin, Adriamycin, cyclophosphamide, Oncovin, dexamethasone
MBC	maximum (maximal) breathing capacity • minimum (minimal) bactericidal concentration
MBD	minimal brain dysfunction
MBF	meat base formula • myocardial blood flow
MBO	management by objectives • mesiobucco-occlusal
MbO$_2$	oxymyoglobin
MBP	mean blood pressure • melitensis, bovine, porcine (antigen) • myelin basic protein (assay)
MBRT	methylene blue reduction time
MBT	mixed bacterial toxin
mc	millicurie
Mc	megacurie • megacycle
MC	macroglobulinemia • Master of Surgery (Magister Chirurgiae) • medical center • medical corps • medullary cystic disease • metacarpal • microencephaly • mineralocorticoid • mixed cellularity • mycelial phase
M&C	morphine and cocaine
M-C	Magovern-Cromie (prosthesis)
MCA	middle cerebral artery
MCAR	mixed-cell agglutination reaction
MCAT	Medical College Admission Test
McB	McBurney's point
MCB	membranous cytoplasmic body
MCCU	Mobile Coronary Care Unit

MCD	mean corpuscular diameter • medullary cystic disease • metabolic coronary dilation
MCE	medical-care evaluation • Medicare Code Editor
MCF	macrophage chemotactic factor • medium corpuscular fragility
mcg	microgram
MCGN	mesangiocapillary glomerulonephritis
mch	millicurie-hour
MCh	Master of Surgery (*Magister Chirurgiae*)
MCH	maternal and child health • mean corpuscular hemoglobin • Microfibrillar Collagen Hemostat
MCHB	Maternal and Child Health Bureau
MCHC	mean corpuscular hemoglobin concentration
MCHS	maternal and child health services
mCi	millicurie
mCid	millicuries destroyed
MCL	maximum containment laboratory • midclavicular line • modified chest lead
MCL$_1$	modified chest lead
MCLNS	mucocutaneous lymph-node syndrome
MCNS	minimal-change nephrotic syndrome
mcoul	millicoulomb
MCP	metacarpal • metaclopramide
MCPH	metacarpophalangeal
mcps	megacycles per second
MCR	metabolic clearance rate
MCT	mean circulation time • medium-chain triglyceride • medullary carcinoma of the thyroid • multiple compressed tablet
MCTD	mixed connective-tissue disease
MCU	maximum care unit

MCV	mean cell volume • mean clinical value • mean corpuscular volume
md	median
Md	mendelevium
MD	Doctor of Medicine *(Medicinae Doctor)* • macular degeneration • mandibular • manic depression • mean deviation • medical department • mentally deficient • mesiodistal • mitral disease • muscular dystrophy
MDA	malonyldialdehyde • manual dilatation of the anus • methylenedioxyamphetamine (hallucinogenic drug) • motor discriminative acuity • Muscular Dystrophy Association • right mentoanterior *(mentodextra anterior)*
MDC	Major Diagnostic Category
MDD	major depressive disorder • mean daily dose
MDF	myocardial depressant factor
MDH	malate dehydrogenase
MDI	metered dose inhaler • multiple daily injections
m dict	as directed *(more dictu)*
Mdn	median
MDP	right mentoposterior *(mentodextra posterior)*
MDQ	minimal detectable quantity
MDR	minimum (minimal) daily requirement
MDS	Master of Dental Surgery • minimal data sheet
MDSO	mentally disordered sex offender
MDT	right mentotransverse *(mentodextra transversa)*
Me	methyl
ME	maximum effort • medical education • medical examiner • metabolic and electrolyte disorder • middle ear
M/E	myeloid-erythroid ratio
MEA	multiple endocrine adenomatosis

meas	measure, measured, measuring
MeB	methylene blue
mec	meconium
MEC	medical executive committee • minimum effective concentration
MeCCNU	semustine
mech	mechanism
med	median • medicine, medical • medium
MED	median erythrocyte diameter • minimum (minimal) effective dose • minimum (minimal) erythema dose
MEDLARS	Medical Literature Analysis and Retrieval System
MEDLINE	MEDLARS on-line
MEDPAR	Medicare Provider Analysis and Review
MEDPRO	Medical Education Resources Program
med-surg	medical-surgical
med tech	medical technician • medical technologist
MEE	methylethyl ether
MEF	maximum (maximal) expiratory flow
MEFR	maximum (maximal) expiratory flow rate
MEFV	maximum (maximal) expiratory flow volume
meg	megacycle • megaloblastic
MEG	mercaptoethylguanidine
MEL	murine erythroleukemia
mem	member
MEM	macrophage electrophoretic migration • macrophage electrophoretic mobility • minimum (minimal) essential medium
memb	membrane
MEN	multiple endocrine neoplasia
menst	menstrual, menstruate, menstruating

MEOS	microsomal ethanol-oxidizing system
MEP	mean effective pressure • motor end-plate
mEq	milliequivalent
mEq/L	milliequivalents per liter
MER	methanol extraction residue
MES	maintenance electrolyte solution • morpholino-ethanesoufonic acid
MESH	Medical Subject Headings
met	metal, metallic
Met	methionine
MET	metabolic equivalent • multiple-employer trust
metab	metabolic, metabolism, metabolites
metas	metastasis, metastasize, metastasizing
meth	method
metHb	methemoglobin
methyl-CCNU	semustine
metMb	metmyoglobin
mets	metastasis, metastasize, metastasizing
m et sig	mix and write a label *(misce et signa)*
mev	megaelectron-volt (million electron-volts)
meV	megaelectron-volt (million electron-volts)
MeV	megaelectron-volt (million electron-volts)
mf	microfilaria
mF	millifarad
MF	medium frequency • microscopic factor • mitotic figure • multiplying factor • mycosis fungoides • myelin figure
M/F	male-female ratio
M&F	male and female • mother and father

MFA	methyl fluoracetate
MFAT	multifocal atrial tachycardia
MFB	medial forebrain bundle • metallic foreign body
MFD	maternal-fetal diagnostics • midforceps delivery • minimum (minimal) fatal dose
MFG	modified heat-degraded gelatin
M flac	*membrana flaccida*
MFP	monofluorophosphate
MFPVC	multifocal premature ventricular contractions
MFS	medical fee schedule
m ft	let a mixture be made *(mistura fiat)*
MFT	muscle-function test
mg	milligram
mg%	milligrams per 100 cubic centimeters or per 100 grams
Mg	magnesium
MG	membranous glomerulopathy • menopausal gonadotrophin • mesiogingival • myasthenia gravis
MGD	mixed gonadal dysgenesis
mg-el	milligram-element
MGF	maternal grandfather
mg-hr	milligram-hour
mg/kg	milligrams per kilogram (of body weight)
mgm	milligram
MGM	maternal grandmother
MgSO$_4$	magnesium sulfate
MH	malignant hyperthermia • marital history • medical history • melanophore hormone • menstrual history • mental health • municipal hospital
MHA	Master in Health Administration • Mental Health Association • microangiopathic hemolytic anemia

MHA-TP	microhemagglutinin-*Treponema pallidum* (test)
MHb	methemoglobin
MHB	maximum (maximal) hospital benefit
MHC	major histocompatibility complex • mental health center • multiphasic health checkup
MHD	maximum (maximal) human dose • minimum (minimal) hemolytic dose
MHI	Mental Health Institute
MHP	maternal health program • mercury hydroxypropane • methoxyhydroxypropane
MHPG	methoxyhydroxyphenylglycol
MHW	mental health worker
MHz	megahertz
MI	maturation index • mental illness • mesioincisal • mitral insufficiency • myocardial infarction
M&I	maternal and infant care
MIA	medically indigent adult • missing in action
MIB	Medical Impairment Bureau
MiC	minocycline
MIC	medical intensive care • microscopic • minimum (minimal) inhibitory concentration • mobile intensive care
MICU	medical intensive care unit • mobile intensive care unit
mid	middle
MID	mesioincisodistal • minimal inhibiting dose • minimum (minimal) infective dose
mid sag	midsagittal
MIF	macrophage-inhibiting factor • melanocyte-inhibiting factor • melanocyte-stimulating hormone-inhibiting factor • merthiolate iodine formalin (solution) • migration-inhibiting factor

MIFR	maximum (maximal) inspiratory flow rate
mil	milliliter
MILIS	Multicenter Investigation of the Limitation of Infarct Size
min	mineral • minim • minimum • minimal • minute • minor
MIO	minimum (minimal) identifiable odor
MIRD	Medical Internal Radiation Dose (Committee)
MIS	Management Information System • medical information services
misc	miscarriage • miscellaneous
mist	mixture *(mistura)*
mit	send *(mitte)*
MIT	Metabolic Intolerance Test • monoiodotyrosine
mit insuf	mitral insufficiency
mIU	milli-international unit
mixt	mixture
MJ	marijuana
MJI	mid-joint injury
MK	marked • monkey kidney
MKM	myopic keratomileusis
MKS	meter-kilogram-second (system)
ml	midline • milliliter
mL	milliliter
ML	Licentiate in Medicine • mesiolingual • middle lobe • midline
MLa	mesiolabial
MLA	left mentoanterior *(mentolaeva anterior)* • Medical Library Association
MLal	mesiolabioincisal
MLaP	mesiolabiopulpal

MLB	mid-line bar
MLBW	moderately low birth weight
MLC	minimum (minimal) lethal concentration • mixed leukocyte culture • mixed lymphocyte culture
MLCR	mixed lymphocyte culture reaction
MLD	masking level differences • median lethal dose • metachromatic leukodystrophy • minimum (minimal) lethal dose
MLEpis	midline episiotomy
MLF	medial longitudinal fasciculus
MLG	mitochondria lipid glucogen
MLI	mesiolinguoincisal
MLNS	mucocutaneous lymph node syndrome
MLO	mesiolinguo-occlusal
MLP	left mentoposterior *(mentolaeva posterior)* • mesiolinguopulpal
MLR	mixed lymphocyte reaction • mixed lymphocyte response
MLS	mean lifespan • median longitudinal section • mucolipidosis
MLT	left mentotransverse *(mentolaeva transversa)* • median lethal time • medical laboratory technician
mm	millimeter • murmur • muscles
mm^2	square millimeter
mm^3	cubic millimeter
mM	millimol (millimole)
MM	medial malleolus • motor meal • mucous membrane • multiple myeloma • myeloid metaplasia
M&M	morbidity and mortality
MMA	methylmalonic acid
MMC	migrating myoelectric complex

MMD	mass median diameter
MME	major movable equipment
MMECT	multiple monitored electroconvulsive therapy
MMEF	maximum (maximal) midexpiratory flow
MMEFR	maximum (maximal) midexpiratory flow rate
MMF	maximum (maximal) midexpiratory flow
MMFR	maximum (maximal) midexpiratory flow rate
mmHg	millimeters of mercury
MMI	methimazole (methylmercaptoimidazole)
MMIS	Medicaid Management Information System
MMK	Marshall-Marchetti-Krantz (procedure)
mM/L	millimols (millimoles) per liter
MMPI	Minnesota Multiphasic Personality Inventory
mmpp	millimeters partial pressure
MMR	mass miniature radiography • mass miniature roentgenography • maternal mortality rate • measles, mumps, rubella • mouth-to-mouth resuscitation
MMS	methyl methanesulfonate
MMSE	Mini Mental State Examination
MMT	manual muscle test
MMTP	methadone maintenance treatment program
MMWR	Morbidity and Mortality Weekly Report
mn	midnight
mN	millinormal
Mn	manganese
MN	midnight • mononuclear • motor neuron • multinodular • myoneural
MNCV	motor-nerve conduction velocity
MND	minimum (minimal) necrotizing dose • motoneuron disease

MNG	multinodular goiter
MNJ	myoneural junction
MNS	minor blood group system
MNU	methylnitrosourea
Mo	mode • molybdenum
MO	manually operated • medical officer • mesio-occlusal • mineral oil • minute output • mitral orifice • month • months old
MOA	mechanisms of allergy • Memorandum of Agreement
MOAB	monoclonal antibody
MOB	medical office building
mod	moderate, moderately • modified • modulation • module
MOD	mesio-occlusodistal • maturity-onset diabetes mellitus
mod praesc	as directed (*modo praescripto*)
MODY	maturity-onset diabetes of youth
MOF	methoxyflurane
MOH	medical officer of health
MOJAC	mood, orientation, judgment, affect, content
mol	molecule, molecular
moll	soft (*mollis*)
mol wt	molecular weight
MOM	milk of magnesia
MoMSV	Moloney murine sarcoma virus
mon	monocyte • month
mono	infectious mononucleosis
monos	monocytes
MOP	medical outpatient program

MOPP	mechlorethamine, Oncovin, procarbazine, prednisone
MOPV	monovalent oral poliovirus vaccine
mor dict	as directed *(more dicto)*
morph	morphology, morphologic
mOs	milliosmol
MOSF	multi-organ system failure
mOsm	milliosmol
m osmole	milliosmol
MOTT	mycobacteria other than tubercle
MOU	memorandum of understanding
mp	as directed *(modo praescripto)* • melting point
MP	mechanical percussion • mechanical percussor • menstrual period • mentoposterior • mercaptopurine • mesiopulpal • metacarpophalangeal • methylprednisolone • monophosphate • mucopolysaccharide
6-MP	6-mercaptopurine
MPA	Master of Public Administration • medroxyprogesterone acetate
MPAP	mean pulmonary artery pressure
MPB	male pattern baldness
MPC	maximum (maximal) permissible concentration
MPCWP	mean pulmonary capillary wedge pressure
MPD	maximum (maximal) permissible dose • myofacial pain dysfunction
MPH	Master of Public Health
MPHR	maximum (maximal) predicted heart rate
MPI	Master Patient Index • maximum point of impulse • multiphasic personality inventory
MPN	most probable number
MPP	maximum (maximal) print position

MPR	mercaptopurine riboside
MPS	macular photocoagulation study • mucopolysaccharide
MPV	mean platelet volume
MQ	memory quotient
mr	milliroentgen
mR	milliroentgen
MR	magnetic resonance • may repeat • measles, rubella • medial rectus • medical record • mental retardation, mentally retarded • metabolic rate • methyl red • milk-ring (test) • mitral reflux • mitral regurgitation • mixed respiratory
MRA	magnetic resonance angiography • Medical Record Administrator
mrad	millirad
MRAN	medical resident admitting note
MRC	Medical Research Council • Medical Reserve Corps
MRCP	Member, Royal College of Physicians
MRCS	Member, Royal College of Surgeons
MRD	minimum (minimal) reacting dose
MRDM	malnutrition-related diabetes mellitus
MRE	maximum (maximal) restrictive exercise
mrem	millirem
MRF	melanocyte-releasing factor • melanocyte-stimulating hormone-releasing factor
MRFIT	multiple risk factor intervention trial
MRH	melanocyte-releasing hormone
MRHD	maximum (maximal) recommended human dose
mrhm	milliroentgens per hour at one meter
MRI	magnetic resonance imaging • mortality risk index
MRIH	melanocyte release-inhibiting hormone

mRNA	messenger ribonucleic acid
MRQ	medical review questionnaire
MRR	marrow release rate
MRS	methicillin-resistant *staphylococcus aureus*
MRSA	methicillin-resistant *staphylococcus aureus*
MRT	major role therapy
MRU	minimum (minimal) reproductive units
MRxi	may repeat one time
ms	millisecond
MS	mass spectrometry • Master of Science • Master of Surgery • medical-surgical • mental status • mitral stenosis • morphine sulfate • multiple sclerosis • muscle strength • musculoskeletal
MSA	Medical Services Administration • Medical Services Association • multiplication stimulating activity
MSD	Master of Science in Dentistry • midsleep disturbance • mild sickle-cell disease • most significant digit • multiple sulfatase deficiency
MSDS	material safety data sheets
MSE	mental status examination
msec	millisecond
MSG	monosodium glutamate
MSH	melanocyte-stimulating hormone • melanophore-stimulating hormone
MSHCA	Master of Science in Health Care Administration
MSHIF	melanocyte-stimulating hormone-inhibiting factor
MSHRF	melanocyte-stimulating hormone-releasing factor
MSL	midsternal line
MSLA	multisample Luer adapter
MSLT	multiple sleep latency test
MSN	Master of Science in Nursing

MSO	management services organization
MSP	Medicare as secondary payor
MSPH	Master of Science in Public Health
MSRPP	Multidimensional Scale for Rating Psychiatric Patients
mss	massage
MSS	medical social services • mental status schedule • metabolic support service • minor surgery suite
MST	median survival time
MSTh	mesothorium
MSU	medical-surgical unit • midstream urine
MSUA	midstream urinalysis
MSUD	maple syrup urine disease
MSV	Moloney's sarcoma virus • murine sarcoma virus
MSW	Master of Social Welfare • Master of Social Work • Medical Social Worker
MT	empty • medial thickening • mediastinal tube • medical technologist, medical technology • metatarsal • music therapy • tympanic membrane *(membrana tympani)*
MT6	mercaptomerin
MT(ASCP)	Registered Medical Technologist (American Society of Clinical Pathologists)
MTBF	mean time between (equipment) failures
MTC	medullary thyroid carcinoma
MTD	maximum (maximal) tolerated dose • metastatic trophoblastic disease
MTF	military treatment facility • modulation transfer function
MTM	modified Thayer-Martin (agar)
MTP	metatarsophalangeal
MTR	Meinicke turbidity reaction
MTT	mean transit time

MTU	methylthiouracil
MTV	mammary tumor virus
MTX	methotrexate
mu	mouse unit
mU	milliunit
Mu	Mache unit
MUGA	multiple-gated acquisition scanning
mult	multiplication, multiply
multip	multipara
MUO	myocardiopathy of unknown origin
MUP	motor unit potential
musc	muscular, muscle
MUST	medical unit, self-contained and transportable
muu	mouse uterine unit
mv	millivolt
mV	millivolt
MV	mechanical ventilation • megavolt • minute volume • mitral valve
MVA	mitral-valve area • motor vehicle accident
MVB	mixed venous blood
MVC	maximum (maximal) vital capacity
MVE	Murray Valley encephalitis
MVI	multivitamin infusion
MVO$_2$	myocardial oxygen consumption • oxygen content of mixed venous blood
MVO$_2$R	myocardial oxygen consumption rate
MVP	mitral valve prolapse
MVPP	Mustargen, vinblastine, procarbazine, prednisone
MVRI	mixed vaccine, respiratory infection

mV-sec	millivolt-second
MVV	maximum (maximal) ventilatory volume • maximum (maximal) voluntary ventilation
MVVPP	Mustargen, vincristine, vinblastine, procarbazine, prednisone
mw	microwave
mW	milliwatt
MW	molecular weight
M-W	Mallory-Weiss syndrome • men and women
MWIA	Medical Women's International Association
MWt	molecular weight
Mx	mastectomy • maxillary • multiple • myringotomy
My	myopia
myco	mycobacterium
myel	myelin • myelogram
myelo	myelocyte
MyG	myasthenia gravis
myo	myocardial, myocardium
MZ	monozygotic, monozygous

N

n	born *(nee)* • nano- (one-billionth) • normal • nostril • number • symbol for index of refraction
N	nasal • negative • *Neisseria* • nerve • neurologist, neurology • neuter • neutron dosage unit • newton • nitrogen • nodal • nonmalignant • normal • normal concentration • number
Na	sodium *(natrium)*
NA	Narcotics Anonymous • neutralizing antibody • nicotinic acid • *Nomina Anatomica* (nomenclature) • noradrenalin (norepinephrine) • not applicable • not available • nuclear antigen • nucleic acid • numeric aperture • nurse anesthetist • nurse's aide • nursing assistant
NAA	no apparent abnormalities
NAACOG	Nurses Association of the American College of Obstetricians and Gynecologists
NAATP	National Association of Addiction Treatment Providers
NaBr	sodium bromide
NAC	*N*-acetylcysteine • Nursing Audit Committee
NACA	National Advisory Council on Aging
NaCl	sodium chloride
NAD	National Association of the Deaf • nicotinamide adenine dinucleotide • nicotinic acid dehydrogenase • no acute distress • no apparent distress • no appreciable disease • nothing abnormal detected

NADH	nicotinamide adenine dinucleotide, reduced form
NADONA/ LTC	National Association of Directors of Nursing Administration in Long Term Care
NADP	nicotinamide adenine dinucleotide phosphate
NADPH	nicotinamide adenine dinucleotide phosphate, reduced form
NaF	sodium fluoride
NAG	nonagglutinable vibrios
NAHC	National Association for Home Care
NaHCO₃	sodium bicarbonate
NAHQ	National Association for Healthcare Quality
NAI	non-accidental injury
NaI(TI)	thallium-activated sodium iodide (scintillation detector)
NALGHC	National Alliance of Lesbian and Gay Health Clinics
NAMH	National Association for Mental Health
NANA	*N*-acetylneuraminic acid
NANAD	National Association of Anorexia Nervosa and Related Disorders
NANB	non-A, non-B (viral hepatitis)
NANBV	non-A, non-B virus
NANDA	North American Nursing Diagnosis Association
NAP	nonacute profile
NAPA	*N*-acetyl-*p*-aminophenol (acetaminophen) • *N*-acetylprocainamide
NAPCA	National Air Pollution Control Administration
NAPNAP	National Association of Pediatric Nurse Associates and Practitioners
NAPNES	National Association for Practical Nurse Education and Service
NAPPH	National Association of Private Psychiatric Hospitals

NAPS	National Auxiliary Publications Service
NAPT	National Association of Physical Therapists
NAQAP	National Association of Quality Assurance Professionals
NAR	nasal airway resistance
NARC	narcotic • narcotics officer • National Association for Retarded Children
NAS	nasal • National Academy of Sciences • no added salt
NASA	National Aeronautics and Space Administration
NASCD	National Association for Sickle Cell Disease
NAS-NRC	National Academy of Sciences - National Research Council
NASW	National Association of Social Workers
nat	national • native • nature, natural
NATCO	North American Transplant Coordinators Organization
Nb	niobium
NB	Negri bodies • newborn • normoblast • note well *(nota bene)*
NBC	nuclear, biological, chemical
NBI	no bone injury
NBM	nothing by mouth
NBME	National Board of Medical Examiners
NBN	Newborn Nursery
NBO	nonbed occupancy
NBR	Nursing Boards Review
NBS	National Bureau of Standards
NBT	nitroblue tetrazolium
NBTE	nonbacterial thrombotic endocarditis
NBTNF	newborn, term, normal, female

NBTNM	newborn, term, normal, male
nc	nanocurie
NC	nasal cannula • no change • noncontributory • nurse corps
N/C	no complaints
NCA	National Certification Agency • National Council on Alcoholism • neurocirculatory asthenia • nonspecific cross-reacting antigen
NcAMP	nephrogenous cyclic adenosine monophosphate
NCB	no code blue
NCCLS	National Committee for Clinical Laboratory Standards
NCCMHC	National Council of Community Mental Health Centers
NCD	not considered disabling
NCF	night care facility
NCHCA	National Commission for Health Certifying Agencies
NCHS	National Center for Health Statistics
NCHSR	National Center for Health Services Research
nCi	nanocurie
NCI	naphthalene creosote, iodoform (powder) • National Cancer Institute
NCLEX	National Council Licensure Examination for Nurses
NCME	Network for Continuing Medical Education
NCN	National Council of Nurses
NCNC	normochromic, normocytic (erythrocyte)
NCNR	National Center for Nursing Research
NCP	National Cancer Program • nursing care plan
NCR	neurologic/circulatory/range of motion
NCRP	National Council on Radiation Protection and Measurements
NCS	noncoronary sinus

NCSH	National Clearinghouse for Smoking and Health
NCSNNE	National Commission for the Study of Nursing and Nursing Education
NCV	noncholera vibrio
NCVS	nerve conduction velocity studies
n$_D$	refractive index
Nd	neodymium
ND	Doctor of Nursing • natural death • neoplastic disease • neutral density • New Drugs (AMA publication) • normal delivery • not diagnosed • not done
NDA	National Dental Association • New Drug Application
NDC	National Drug Code (number)
NDCD	National Drug Code Directory
NDE	near-death experience
NDF	no disease found
NDGA	nordihydroguaiaretic acid
NDM	*N*-desmethylmethsuximide
NDT	Neurological Development Therapy • non-destructive testing
NDTI	National Disease and Therapeutic Index
NDV	Newcastle Disease Virus
NDx	nondiagnostic
Nd:YAG	neodymium: yttrium aluminum garnet (laser)
Ne	neon
NE	neurological examination • no ectopy • norepinephrine • not enlarged • not examined • nursing educator
neb	nebulizer
NEC	necrotizing enterocolitis • not elsewhere classified
NED	no evidence of disease • normal equivalent deviation

NEEP	negative end-expiratory pressure
NEF	Nurses Educational Fund
NEFA	nonesterified fatty acid
neg	negative
NEISS	National Electronic Injury Surveillance System
neo	neoarsphenamine
NEP	negative expiratory pressure
NER	nonionizing electromagnetic radiation
nerv	nervous
neuro	neurologic
NF	National Formulary • none found • nonfunction • normal flow
NFCC	neighborhood family-care center
NFIC	National Foundation for Ileitis and Colitis
NFLPN	National Federation for Licensed Practical Nurses
NFP	natural family planning • not for profit
NFPA	National Fire Protection Association
NFSID	National Foundation for Sudden Infant Death
NFTD	normal, full-term delivery
ng	nanogram
NG	nasogastric • new growth • no good
NGF	nerve growth factor
NGR	narrow gauze roll
NGS	National Geriatrics Society
NGT	nasogastric tube
NGU	nongonococcal urethritis
NH	nodal-His • nodular and histiocytic • nursing home
NH$_3$	ammonia
NH$_4$+	ammonium ion

NH4Cl	ammonium chloride
NHF	National Hemophilia Foundation
NHI	national health insurance • National Heart Institute
NHIF	National Head Injury Foundation
NHL	non-Hodgkin's lymphoma
NHLBI	National Heart, Lung and Blood Institute
NHLI	National Heart and Lung Institute
NHPP	normal human pooled plasma
NHS	National Health Service • normal human serum
NHSC	National Health Service Corps
Ni	nickel
NIA	National Institute on Aging • no information available
NIAA	National Institute on Alcohol Abuse and Alcoholism
NIADDK	National Institute of Arthritis, Diabetes and Digestive and Kidney Diseases
NIAID	National Institute of Allergy and Infectious Diseases
NIAMD	National Institute of Arthritis and Metabolic Diseases
NICHE	Nurses Improving Care to the Hospitalized Elderly
NICHHD	National Institute of Child Health and Human Development
NICU	neonatal intensive care unit • newborn intensive care unit
NIDA	National Institute on Drug Abuse
NIDDKD	National Institute of Diabetes, Digestive & Kidney Diseases
NIDDM	noninsulin-dependent diabetes mellitus
NIDR	National Institute of Dental Research
NIEHS	National Institute of Environmental Health Services
NiF	negative inspiratory force
NIGMS	National Institute of General Medical Sciences

NIH	National Institutes of Health
NIHD	noise-induced hearing damage
NIMH	National Institute of Mental Health
NINCDS	National Institute of Neurological and Communicative Disorders and Stroke
NINDB	National Institute of Neurological Diseases and Blindness
NINDS	National Institute of Neurological Diseases and Stroke
NIOSH-CDC	National Institute for Occupational Safety and Health - Centers for Disease Control
NIP	National Inpatient Profile
NIRMP	National Interns and Residents Matching Program
NIRR	noninsulin-requiring remission
NIT	nasointestinal tube
nit ox	nitrous oxide
NJPC	National Joint Practice Commission
NK	natural killer (cells)
NKA	no known allergies
NKDA	no known drug allergies
NKF	National Kidney Foundation
nl	nanoliter
NL	normal
NLA	neuroleptanalgesia
NLM	National Library of Medicine
NLN	National League for Nursing
NLP	neurolinguistic program • no light perception
NLT	not later than • not less than
nm	nanometer
nM	nanomolar

NM	neuromuscular • night and morning • nitrogen mustard • nodular and mixed (lymphocytic-histiocytic) • nuclear medicine
NMC	nodular, mixed-cell (lymphoma) • Nurse Managed Center
NMHA	National Mental Health Association
NMI	no middle initial
NMM	nodular malignant melanoma
NMN	nicotinamide mononucleotide • no middle name
nmol	nanomol (nanomole)
NMR	nuclear magnetic resonance
NMRI	Naval Medical Research Institute
NMRS	National Registry of Medical Secretaries
NMS	neuroleptic malignant syndrome
NMSS	National Multiple Sclerosis Society
nn	nerves
NN	nurses' notes
N:N	azo group (chemical group with two nitrogen atoms)
NND	neonatal death • New and Nonofficial Drugs (AMA publication)
NNE	neonatal necrotizing enterocolitis
NNN	Nicolle-Novy-MacNeal (medium)
NNP	neonatal nurse practitioner
NNR	New and Nonofficial Remedies
NNS	non-nutritive sucking
no	number *(numero)*
No	nobelium
NO	nitric oxide • nitroso- • nursing office
N$_2$O	nitrous oxide
NOA	notice of admission

NOAADN	National Organization for the Advancement of Associate Degree Nursing
noc	night *(nox)*
NOCA	National Organization for Competency Assurance
noct	at night *(nocte)*
noct maneq	at night and in the morning *(nocte maneque)*
NODSS	nasal/oral discriminate sampling system
NOFTT	nonorganic failure to thrive
NOMI	nonocclusive mesenteric infarction
non rep	do not repeat *(non repetatur)*
NOP	National Outpatient Profile
NOPHN	National Organization for Public Health Nursing
norm	normal
normet	normetanephrine
NOS	not otherwise specified
NOTT	nocturnal oxygen therapy trial
Np	neptunium
NP	neuropeptide • neuropsychiatric • not otherwise provided for • nucleoplasmic index • nucleoprotein • nurse-practitioner • nursing procedure
NPA	National Perinatal Association • near point of accommodation • no previous admission
NPC	nasopharyngeal carcinoma • near point of convergence • nodal premature contraction • nonproductive cough • no previous complaint
NPCN	National Poison Center Network
NPD	Niemann-Pick disease • nonprescription drugs
NPDB	National Practitioner Data Bank
NPDR	nonproliferative diabetic retinopathy

NPH	neutral protamine Hagedorn (insulin) • no previous history • normal-pressure hydrocephalus
NPJT	nonparoxysmal junctional tachycardia
NPN	nonprotein nitrogen
npo	nothing by mouth *(nulla per os)*
npo/hs	nothing by mouth at bedtime *(nulla per os hora somni)*
NPP	non-physician provider • nurse in private practice
NPR	Notice of Program Reimbursement
NPRM	notice of proposed rule-making
NPSG	nocturnal polysomnogram
NPSRC	National Professional Standards Review Council
NPT	normal pressure and temperature
nr	do not repeat *(non repetatur)*
NR	nerve root • neutral red • nonreactive • non-rebreathing • no refill • normal range • normal record
NRB	non-reportable birth
NRBC	nucleated red blood cells
NRC	National Research Council • noise reduction coefficient • normal retinal correspondence • Nuclear Regulatory Commission
NRC-NAS	National Research Council - National Academy of Sciences
NREM	nonrapid eye movement, non-REM sleep
NRMC	Naval Regional Medical Center
NRMS	National Registry of Medical Secretaries
nRNA	nuclear ribonucleic acid
NRS	normal rabbit serum
ns	nanosecond • no sequelae • nylon suture

NS	nephrotic syndrome • nervous system • neurosurgery, neurosurgical, neurosurgeon • nodular sclerosis • normal saline • normal serum • not significant • not stated • Nursing Services
1/2 NS	half-normal saline
NSA	Neurological Society of America • normal serum albumin • no significant abnormality • nursing service administration
NSABP	National Surgical Adjuvant Breast Project
NSAC	National Society for Autistic Children
NSAID	nonsteroidal anti-inflammatory drug
NSC	non service-connected
NSCC	National Society for Crippled Children
NSCIF	National Spinal Cord Injury Foundation
NSCLC	non-small cell lung cancer
NS/CST	nipple stimulation/contraction stress test
NSD	nitrogen-specific detector • nominal standard dose • normal spontaneous delivery • no significant defect • no significant deficiency
nsec	nanosecond
NSF	National Science Foundation
NSFTD	normal spontaneous full-term delivery
nsg	nursing
NSGCT	nonsiminomatous germ cell tumors
NSHD	nodular sclerosing Hodgkin's disease
NSIDSF	National Sudden Infant Death Syndrome Foundation
NSILA	nonsuppressible insulin-like activity
NSILP	nonsuppressible insulin-like protein
NSNA	National Student Nurses' Association
NSP	not specified
NSPB	National Society for the Prevention of Blindness

NSR	normal sinus rhythm
NSS	normal saline solution • nutritional support services
NSST	Northwestern Syntax Screening Test
NST	naso-tracheal • nonstress test • not sooner than • nutrition support team
NSU	nonspecific urethritis
NSVD	normal spontaneous vaginal delivery
nsy	nursery
NT	nasotracheal • neutralization test • not tested
N&T	nose and throat
NTA	Narcotics Treatment Administration • National Tuberculosis Association
N/TBC	nontuberculous
NTBR	not to be resuscitated
NTD	neural tube defect
NTG	nitroglycerin
NTMI	nontransmural myocardial infarction
NTP	nitropaste • normal temperature and pressure
NTV	nervous tissue vaccine
nU	nanounit
nuc	nucleated
nucl	nuclear
NUD	nonulcer dyspepsia
NUG	necrotizing ulcerative gingivitis
Nullip	nulliparous
num	numerator
NUN	non-urea nitrogen
NV	naked vision • near vision • next visit • nonvaccinated • non-venereal • non-volatile
N&V	nausea and vomiting

NVD	nausea, vomiting, diarrhea • neck-venous distention • nonvalvular (heart) disease • no venous distention
NVWSC	nonvolatile whole-smoke condensate
NW	naked weight
NWB	nonweight-bearing
NYD	not yet diagnosed
NYHA	New York Heart Association (classification)
NYP	not yet published
nyst	nystagmus
NZB	New Zealand black (mouse)
NZW	New Zealand white (mouse)

O

o	ortho
O	doctor's office • eye *(oculus)* • none • occiput, occipital • oral, orally • orthopedic • other • output • oxygen • pint *(octarius)*
O̅	without
O$_2$	both eyes • oxygen
O$_3$	ozone
OA	occiput anterior • ocular albinism • old age • orotic acid • osteoarthritis • oxalic acid • oxaloacetic acid
OAA	Old Age Assistance • oxaloacetic acid
OAAD	ovarian ascorbic acid depletion (test)
OAF	open air factor • osteoclast- activating factor • osteocyte- activation factor
OALF	organic acid-labile fluoride
OAP	ophthalmic artery pressure
OASDHI	Old Age-Survivors Disability and Health Insurance
OASI	Old Age and Survivors Insurance
OASP	organic acid-soluble phosphorus
OAVD	oculoauriculovertebral dysplasia
OB	obstetric(s), obstetrician • occult blood
OBG	obstetrician-gynecologist • obstetrics and gynecology
OB/GYN	obstetrician-gynecologist • obstetrics and gynecology
obl	oblique
OBRA	Omnibus Budget Reconciliation Act (1986)

OBS	organic brain syndrome
obsd	observed
obst	obstetric(s), obstetrician • obstruction
OC	occlusocervical • office call • only child • oral contraceptive • oxygen consumed
O&C	onset and course
OCA	oral contraceptive agent
O₂Cap	oxygen capacity
occ	occasional • occiput, occipital
occas	occasional, occasionally
OCD	obsessive-compulsive disorder • ovarian cholesterol depletion
OCE	other controllable expenses
OCG	oral cholecystogram
OCN	Oncology Certified Nurse
O₂Con	oxygen concentration • oxygen content
OCP	oral contraceptive pills • ova, cysts and parasites
OCT	oral contraceptive therapy • ornithine carbamoyltransferase • oxytocin challenge test
O₂CT	oxygen content
OCU	observation care unit • outpatient care unit
OCV	ordinary conversational voice
od	every day (*omni die*)
OD	Doctor of Optometry • occupational disease • Officer of the Day • once daily • open drop • optical density • outside diameter • overdose • right eye (*oculus dexter*)
ODA	right occipitoanterior (*occipitodextra anterior*)
ODC	oxygen dissociation curve • oxyhemoglobin dissociation curve
ODP	right occipitoposterior (*occipitodextra posterior*)

ODT	right occipitotransverse *(occipitodextra transversa)*
OE	on examination • otitis externa
OEE	outer enamel epithelium
O&E	observation and examination
O/E	ratio of observed to expected
OEM	open-end marriage
OEO	Office of Economic Opportunity
OER	oxygen-enhancement ratio
OERR	order entry and results reporting
OF	occipitofrontal • other facility
OFD	object-to-film distance • occipitofrontal diameter • oral-facial-digital (syndrome)
off	official
OFTT	organic failure to thrive
OG	orogastric
OGA	orogastric aspirate
OGTT	oral glucose tolerance test
oh	every hour *(omni hora)*
OH	hydroxyl group • occupational health • open-heart • orthostatic hypotension • out-patient hospital
OHC	outer hair cell
OHCS	hydroxycorticosteroid
OHD	organic heart disease
OHF	Omsk hemorrhagic fever • overhead frame
OHFA	hydroxy fatty acids
OHI	ocular hypertension indicator
ohm-cm	ohm-centimeter
OHP	hydroxyproline • oxygen under high pressure
OHS	occupational health service • open-heart surgery

OHT	over-head trapeze
OI	opportunistic infection • opsonic index • osteogenesis imperfecta • oxygen intake
OIH	ortho-iodohippurate • ovulation-inducing hormone
oint	ointment
OJ	orange juice
OJT	on-the-job training
OKN	optokinetic nystagmus
Ol	oil
OL	left eye *(oculus laevus)*
OLA	left occipitoanterior *(occipitolaeva anterior)*
OLB	open lung biopsy
Ol oliv	olive oil *(oleum olivae)*
OLP	left occipitoposterior *(occipitolaeva posterior)*
OLT	left occipitotransverse *(occipitolaeva transversa)* • orthotopic liver transplantation
om	every morning *(omni mane)*
OM	occipitomental (diameter of head) • Occupational Medicine • osteomyelitis • otitis media
OMA	Office of Medical Affairs
OMB	Office of Management and Budget
OME	otitis media with effusion
OML	orbitomeatal line
omn bih	every two hours *(omni bihora)*
omn hor	every hour *(omni hora)*
omn noct	every night *(omni nocte)*
OMPA	octamethyl pyrophosphoramide
OMVI	operating a motor vehicle intoxicated
on	every night *(omni nocte)*
ON	optic neuritis

onco	oncology
OND	other neurological disease
ONP	operating nursing procedure
OOA	out-of-area
OOB	out of bed
OOF	owned and operated facility
OOLR	ophthalmology, otology, laryngology, and rhinology
OOT	out of town
OP	occipitoparietal • occipitoposterior • opening pressure • operative procedure • orthopedic condition • osmotic pressure • outpatient
O&P	ova and parasites
OPA	organ procurement agency
OPB	outpatient basis
OPC	outpatient clinic
op cit	in the work cited *(opere citato)*
OPD	optical path difference • outpatient department • outpatient dispensary
opg	opening
OPG	oculoplethysmography
Oph	ophthalmology • ophthalmoscope
Ophth	ophthalmology • ophthalmoscope
OpMi	operating microscope
OPO	organ procurement organization
opp	opposite • opposed
OPS	outpatient section • outpatient service • outpatient surgery
OPSC	outpatient surgery center
OPSR	Office of Professional Standards Review
opt	optical, optician, optics • optimal

OPT	outpatient
OPV	oral poliovirus vaccine
OQS	Office of Quality Standards
o/r	oxidation/reduction
OR	occupancy rate • oil retention enema • operating room • organ recovery • orienting reflex
O-R	oxidation-reduction
ORC	order/results/communication
ord	orderly • ordinate
ORD	optical rotatory dispersion
OREF	open reduction external fixation
OR en	oil retention enema
org	organic • organism
ORG	optimal recovery guidelines
ORH	Office of Rural Health
ORIF	open reduction internal fixation
orig	origin, original
ORL	otorhinolaryngology
ORN	Operating Room Nurse
ORS	Orthopedic Research Society • orthopedic surgery
ORT	operating room technician
orth	orthopedics
ortho	orthopedics
ORx	oriented
os	mouth (*os*)
Os	osmium
OS	left eye (*oculus sinister*) • Osgood-Schlatter's disease • osteogenic sarcoma
OSA	obstructive sleep apnea

OSAS	obstructive sleep apnea syndrome
O₂Sat	oxygen saturation
osc	oscillate
OSD	overside drainage
OSHA	Occupational Safety and Health Administration
osm	osmol
OSMF	oral submucous fibrosis
OST	Office of Science and Technology
osteo	osteomyelitis
OT	objective test • occipitotransverse • occupational therapist, occupational therapy • old terminology • old tuberculin • oral thrush • orotracheal • otolaryngology, otolaryngologist
OTA	Office of Technology Assessment
OTC	ornithine transcarbamylase • over-the-counter • oxytetracycline
OTCD	over-the-counter drug
OTCRx	over-the-counter drug
OTD	organ tolerance dose
oto	otology, otologist
otol	otology, otologist
OTR	Registered Occupational Therapist
OTSG	Office of the Surgeon General
OU	both eyes *(oculi unitas)* • each eye *(oculus uterque)* • observation unit
ov	egg *(ovum)* • ovary
OV	obvious • office visit
OVD	occlusal vertical dimension
OW	out-of-wedlock
O/W	oil in water

oxidn	oxidation
OXT	oxytocin
oz	ounce *(onza)*
oz. ap.	ounces apothecary's
oz. av.	ounces avoirdupois

P

p	after *(post)* • by weight *(pondere)* • handful *(pugillus)* • near *(proximum)* • papilla • para- • partial pressure • pico- • probable error • pupil
P	by weight *(pondere)* • para- • parenteral • part • partial pressure • pharmacopeia • phenolphthalein • phosphorus • pico- • pint • plasma • pole • population • position • positive • posterior • postpartum • presbyopia • pressure • probable error • protein • psoralen • psychiatrist, psychiatry • pulse • pupil
p̄	after *(post)* • mean pressure (gas)
P₁	first parental generation • pulmonic first sound
P₂	pulmonic second sound
³²P	radioactive phosphorus • radiophosphorus
Pa	Pascal (unit of pressure) • protactinium
PA	panic attack • paralysis agitans • parietal cell antibody • pathology • permeability area • pernicious anemia • phosphoarginine • physician advisor • physician's assistant • plasminogen activator • posteroanterior • primary amenorrhea • primary anemia • procainamide • professional association • prolonged action • proprietary association • protrusio acetabuli • psycho-analysis, psychoanalyst • pulmonary artery • pulpoaxial
P&A	percussion and auscultation
PAB	para-aminobenzoic (acid) • premature atrial beat
PABA	para-aminobenzoic acid
PAC	papular acrodermatitis of childhood • parent-adult-child • phenacetin,aspirin, caffeine • pre-admission certification • premature atrial contraction

PACE	performance and cost efficiency
PaCO$_2$	arterial carbon dioxide partial pressure • partial pressure of carbon dioxide
PACO$_2$	alveolar carbon dioxide partial pressure
PACU	Post-Anesthesia Care Unit
PAD	per adjusted discharge • phenacetin, aspirin, desoxyephedrine
p ae	in equal parts *(partes aequales)*
PAEDP	pulmonary artery end-diastolic pressure
PAF	platelet-activating factor • platelet-aggregating factor • pulmonary arteriovenous fistula
PAH	para-aminohippuric (acid)
PAHA	para-aminohippuric acid
PAIg	platelet-associated immunoglobulin
PAL	pediatric advanced life support • posterior axillary line
palp	palpable
PALS	periarteriolar lymphocyte sheaths
PA-LS-ID	pernicious anemia-like syndrome and immunoglobulin deficiency
Palv	alveolar pressure
PAM	crystalline penicillin G in aluminum monostearate • phenylalanine mustard • pralidoxime • pulmonary alveolar microlithiasis
PAMP	pulmonary artery mean pressure
PAN	periarteritis nodosa • peroxyacetyl nitrate • polyarteritis nodosa
pancreat	pancreatic
PAO	patient assessment office • peak acid output • psychiatric admitting office
PaO$_2$	arterial oxygen partial pressure • partial pressure of oxygen

PAO$_2$	alveolar oxygen partial pressure • oxygen content of pulmonary artery blood
PAOP	pulmonary artery occlusion pressure
pap	papilla
Pap	papanicolaou (smear, stain, test)
PAP	patient assessment procedure • peroxidase-antiperoxidase (method) • primary atypical pneumonia • private ambulatory patient • prostatic acid phosphatase • pulmonary alveolar proteinosis • pulmonary artery pressure
par	parallel
PAr	polyarteritis
PAR	postanesthesia recovery • postanesthesia room • problem-analysis report
para	a woman who has given birth • number of pregnancies producing viable offspring: para-0, para-I, para-II, etc.
paradox	paradoxical
par aff	part affected
PARP	poly-ADP-ribose polymerase
PARS	Personal Adjustment and Role Skills Scale
part aeq	in equal parts (*partes aequales*)
part vic	in divided doses (*partitis vicibus*)
PARU	postanesthesia recovery unit
Pas	pascal (unit of pressure)
PAS	para-aminosalicylic (acid) • patient appointment and scheduling • performance appraisal system • periodic acid-Schiff (method, reaction, stain, technique, test) • pre-admission screening • pregnancy advisory service • professional activities study
PASA	para-aminosalicylic acid
PAS-C	para-aminosalicylic acid crystallized with ascorbic acid

PASG	pneumatic anti-shock garment
PASP	pulmonary artery systolic pressure
Past	*Pasteurella*
pat	patent • patient
PAT	paroxysmal atrial tachycardia • pre-admission testing • pregnancy at term
path	pathologist, pathology, pathologic
PATH	Partnership Approach to Health
PAVe	procarbazine, melphalen, vinblastine
PAWP	pulmonary artery wedge pressure
Pb	lead *(plumbum)*, presbyopia
PB	Paul-Bunnell (antibodies, test) • peripheral blood • Pharmacopoeia Britannica • phonetically balanced • pinch biopsy • pressure breathing
PBA	percutaneous bladder aspiration
PBB	polybrominated biphenyl
PBC	point of basal convergence • primary biliary cirrhosis
PBE	a form of tuberculin *(Perlsucht bacillen emulsion)*
PBG	porphobilinogen
PBI	protein-bound iodine
PBL	peripheral-blood lymphocytes
PBP	porphyrin biosynthetic pathway • progressive bulbar palsy
PBS	peripheral-blood smear • phosphate-buffered saline • polybrominated salicylanilides
PBSCT	peripheral blood stem cell transplantation
PBV	pulmonary blood volume
PBW	posterior bite wing
PBZ	Pyribenzamine
pc	after meals *(post cibos)* • per cent • picocurie

PC	avoirdupois weight *(pondus civile)* • packed cells • parent cell • parent to child • personal computer • phosphatidylcholine • phosphocreatine • platelet concentrate • platelet count • pneumotoxic center • presenting complaint • professional corporation • pubococcygeus • pulmonary capillary
PCA	patient controlled analgesia • passive cutaneous anaphylaxis • personal care attendant
PCAST	President's Committee of Advisers on Science and Technology
Pcb	near point of convergence to the intercentral baseline
PCB	paracervical block
PCBs	polychlorinated biphenyls
PCc	periscopic concave
PCC	patient-care coordinator • pheochromocytoma • phosphate-carrier compound • Poison Control Center
PCD	polycystic disease
PCF	Patient Compensation Fund • pharyngoconjunctival fever • prothrombin conversion factor
PCG	phonocardiogram, phonocardiography
PCH	paroxysmal cold hemoglobinuria
PCi	picocurie
PCI	pneumatosis cystoides intestinorum
PCK	polycystic kidney (disease)
PCM	patient case manager • protein-calorie malnutrition
PCMR	President's Committee on Mental Retardation
PCN	penicillin • primary care network, nurse
PCNG	penicillin-G
PCNL	percutaneous nephrostolithotomy
PCO	patient complains of
pCO$_2$	partial pressure of carbon dioxide

PCO$_2$	partial pressure of carbon dioxide
PCP	peripheral coronary pressure • phenylcyclidine (hallucinogenic drug) • *Pneumocystis carinii* pneumonia • Primary Care Physician • Psilcybin
PCPA	para-chlorophenylalanine
pcpt	perception
PCr	phosphocreatine
PCR	polymerase chain reaction • probable causal relationship
pcs	preconscious
PCS	patient-care standards • patient-care systems • patient classification system • primary C-section
PCT	plasmacrit test • porcine calcitonin • porphyria cutanea tarda • prothrombin consumption test • proximal convoluted tubule
PCU	patient-care unit (of cost) • progressive care unit
p cut	percutaneous
PCV	packed-cell volume • parietal-cell vagotomy • polycythemia vera
PCW	pulmonary capillary wedge
PCWP	pulmonary capillary wedge pressure
PCx	periscopic convex
PCXR	portable chest x-ray
pd	papilla diameter • prism diopter • pupillary distance
PD	Doctor of Pharmacy • interpupillary distance • paralyzing dose • Parkinsonian dementia • Parkinson's disease • pediatrics • peritoneal dialysis • postural drainage • potential difference • pressor dose • prism diopter • provocation dose • psychotic dementia • psychotic depression • pulmonary disease
PD$_{50}$	median paralyzing dose
PDA	patent ductus arteriosus • pediatric allergy

PDB	para-dichlorobenzene
PDC	pediatric cardiology • physical dependence capacity • private diagnostic clinic • pulmonary diffusion capacity
PDE	paroxysmal dyspnea on exertion • prenatally drug exposed
PDF	probability density function
PDGF	platelet-derived growth factor
PDH	packaged disaster hospital • past dental history
PDLL	poorly differentiated lymphocytic lymphoma
PDM	polymyositis and dermatomyositis
PDN	private duty nurse
PDQ	Prescreening Development Questionnaire
pdr	powder
PDR	Physicians' Desk Reference
PDS	pain dysfunction syndrome
PDT	phenyldimethyltriazine • photodynamic therapy
PDW	platelet distribution width
Pe	perylene • pressure on expiration
PE	paper electrophoresis • pharyngoesophageal • phenylephrine • phosphatidylethanolamine • physical examination • physical exercise • plasma exchange • polyethylene • probable error • pulmonary embolism
PEA	pulseless electrical activity
PEC	patient education coordinator • peritoneal exudate cells
Pecho	prostatic echogram
PED	pediatrics, pediatrician
Peds	pediatrics
PEEP	positive end-expiratory pressure • protein electrophoresis

PEF	peak expiratory flow
PEFR	peak expiratory flow rate
PEFV	partial expiratory flow volume
PEG	percutaneous endoscopic gastrostomy • pneumoencephalogram, pneumoencephalography • polyethylene glycol
PEI	phosphorous excretion index
Pel	elastic recoil pressure of lung
PEL	permissible exposure limits
PEM	protein-energy malnutrition
PEMA	phenylethylmalonamide
pen	penetrating • penicillin
PEN	parenteral and enteral nutrition • professional excellence in nursing
PENG	photoelectric nystagmography
Pent	Pentothal
PEP	Performance Evaluation Procedure • phosphoenolpyruvate • polyestradiol phosphate • pre-ejection period • pre-ejection phase
PEP/LVET	pre-ejection period/left ventricular ejection time
PEPR	precision encoder and pattern recognizer
per	periodic • person • through, by *(per)*
PER	pediatric emergency room
perf	perforation, perforating
perim	perimeter
periph	peripheral
PERL	pupils equal and react to light
perm	permanent
perp	perpendicular
PERRLA	pupils equal, round, react to light and accommodation

pers	personal
PERT	Program Evaluation Review Technique
pes	foot *(pes)*
PET	positron emission tomography • pre-eclamptic toxemia • Psychiatric Emergency Team
PETN	pentaerythritol tetranitrate
PETT	positron emission transaxial tomography
pev	peak electron-volts
peV	peak electron-volts
pf	power factor
Pf	permeability factor
PF	physicians' forum • platelet factor • precursor fluid
PFC	persistent fetal circulation • plaque-forming cells
PFFD	proximal femur focal deficiency
PFG	peak-flow gauge
PFK	phosphofructokinase
PFM	peak flowmeter
PFO	patent foramen ovale
PFR	peak flow rate • pericardial friction rub
PFT	pulmonary function test
PFU	plaque-forming unit
pg	picogram
Pg	pregnant
PG	paregoric • pepsinogen • phosphatidylglycerol • pituitary gonadotropin • plasma gastrin • postgraduate • prostaglandin
2-PG	2-phosphoglycerate
3-PG	3-phosphoglycerate
PGA	pteroylglutamic acid
PG-AC	phenylglycine acid chloride

PGB	prostaglandin B
PGE$_2$	prostaglandin E$_2$
PGF	paternal grandfather
PGF$_2\alpha$	prostaglandin F2α
PGH	pituitary growth hormone • plasma growth hormone
PGI2	prostacyclin (prostaglandin I$_2$)
PGM	paternal grandmother
PGO	pontogeniculo-occipital
PGR	psychogalvanic response
PGU	postgonococcal urethritis
PGY	postgraduate year
ph	phase
pH	measure of hydrogen ion concentration (degree of alkalinity or acidity)
Ph	pharmacopoeia • phenanthrene • phenyl • Philadelphia chromosome • phosphate
Ph^1	Philadelphia chromosome
PH	past history • perianal herpes simplex virus infection • personal history • Pharmaceutical Services • pinhole • previous history • public health • pulmonary hypertension
PHA	passive hemagglutination • phenylalanine • phytohemagglutinin
phar	pharmacy, pharmaceutical, pharmacist, pharmacopeia
pharm	pharmacy, pharmaceutical, pharmacist, pharmacopeia
pharmacol	pharmacologic
Pharm B	Bachelor of Pharmacy (*Pharmaciae Baccalaureus*)
Pharm C	Pharmaceutical Chemist
Pharm D	Doctor of Pharmacy (*Pharmaciae Doctor*)
Pharm G	Graduate in Pharmacy
Pharm M	Master of Pharmacy (*Pharmaciae Magister*)

Ph B	Pharmacopoeia Britannica
PHC	post-hospital care • premolar aplasia, hyperhydrosis and premature canities • primary hepatocellular carcinoma
PhD	doctoral degree (Doctor of Philosophy)
PHDD	personal history of depressive disorders
Phe	phenylalanine
PHE	periodic health examination
PHF	paired helical filaments
PhG	German Pharmacopeia • Graduate in Pharmacy
pHi	gastric intramural pH
phial	bottle *(phiala)*
PHKC	postmortem human kidney cells
PHLA	post-heparin lipolytic activity
PHN	public health nurse • public health nursing
PHO	physician-hospital organization
phos	phosphatase • phosphate
PHP	phosphorus • prepaid health plan • pseudohypoparathyroidism
PHPPD	productive hours per patient day
PHS	Public Health Service
PHT	peroxide hemolysis test • phenytoin
PHTN	portal hypertension
phy	phytohemagglutinin
phys	physical • physician
physio	physiologic
Pi.	pressure of inspiration
PI	parainfluenza (virus) • paternity index • performance indicator • present illness • pressure on inspiration • protamine insulin • protease inhibitor

PICC	peripherally inserted central catheter
PICU	pediatric intensive care unit • pulmonary intensive care unit
PID	pelvic inflammatory disease • prolapsed intervertebral disc
PIE	pulmonary infiltration with eosinophilia • pulmonary interstitial emphysema
PIF	peak inspiratory flow • prolactin-inhibiting (inhibitory) factor • proliferation inhibitory factor
PIFR	peak inspiratory flow rate
PIGPA	pyruvate, inosine, glucose, phosphate, adenine
PIH	pregnancy-induced hypertension
pil	pill *(pilula)*
PIN	personal identification number
PINS	person in need of supervision
PINV	post-imperative negativity (reaction)
PIP	peak inspiratory pressure • periodic interim payment • personal injury protection • proximal interphalangeal
PI-PB	performance versus intensity function for phonetically balanced words
pit	pituitary
PITR	plasma iron turnover rate
PIV	parainfluenza virus
PIVKA	protein in vitamin K absence
PJC	premature junctional contraction
PJRT	permanent junctional reciprocating tachycardia
PJS	Peutz-Jeghers syndrome
PJT	paroxysmal junctional tachycardia
PJVT	paroxysmal junctional-ventricular tachycardia
pK	dissociation constant

PK	Prausnitz-Küstner (reaction) • psychokineses • pyruvate kinase
pKa	measure of acid strength
PKF	phagocytosis and killing function
PKS	pharmacokinetic service
PKU	phenylketonuria
Pl	plasma
PL	perception of light • phospholipid • platelet
PL	transpulmonary pressure
PLA	peroxidase-labeled antibodies (test) • pulpolinguoaxial
Plat	platelet
PLDH	plasma lactic dehydrogenase
PLE	polymorphous light eruption
PLED	periodic lateralized epileptiform discharge
PLG	plasminogen
PLISSIT	Permission, Limited Information, Specific Suggestions, Intensive Therapy
PLL	prolymphocytic leukemia
PLM	polarized-light microscope
PLN	posterior lymph node
PLS	primary lateral sclerosis
PLT	platelet • psittacosis-lymphogranuloma venereum-trachoma
plx	plexus
pm	after noon (*post meridiem*) • picometer
pM	picomolar
Pm	promethium

PM	after noon *(post meridiem)* • pacemaker • peritoneal macrophage • petit mal (epilepsy) • physical medicine • pneumo-mediastinum • polymyositis • postmortem • presystolic murmur • preventive medicine • pulpomesial • purple membrane
P/M	parent-metabolite ratio
PMA	papillary, marginal, attached • paramethoxyamphetamine (hallucinogenic drug) • Primary Mental Abilities (test) • progressive muscular atrophy
PMB	polymorphonuclear basophilic (leukocytes) • postmenopausal bleeding
PMC	Patient Management Categories • pseudomembranous colitis
PMD	private medical doctor
PME	polymorphonuclear eosinophilic (leukocytes)
PMF	progressive massive fibrosis
PMH	past medical history • public mental hospital
PMI	past medical illness • patient medication instruction (sheets) • point of maximum (maximal) impulse • point of maximum (maximal) intensity • previous medical illness
PML	progressive multifocal leukoencephalopathy
PMLE	polymorphous light eruption
PMMA	polymethyl methacrylate
PMN	polymorphonuclear neutrophilic (leukocytes) • polymorphonuclear neutrophils
PMNR	periadenitis mucosa necrotica recurrens
PMP	pervious menstrual period
PMPM	per member per month
PMR	physical medicine and rehabilitation • polymyalgia rheumatica • proportionate mortality ratio • proton magnetic resonance
PM&R	physical medicine and rehabilitation

PMS	postmenopausal syndrome • pregnant mare serum • premenstrual syndrome
PMSG	pregnant mare serum gonadotropin
PMT	premenstrual tension
PMVL	posterior mitral-valve leaflet
PN	parenteral nutrition • percussion note • periarteritis nodosa • peripheral nerve • peripheral neuropathy • plaque neutralizing • practical nurse • progress note • psychiatry-neurology • psychoneurology • psychoneurotic, psychoneurosis • pulmonary disease
P&N	psychiatry and neurology
PNA	pentosenucleic acid • peptide nucleic acid
PNC	penicillin • peripheral nucleated cell • premature nodal contraction
PNCM	professional nurse case manager
PND	paroxysmal nocturnal dyspnea • postnasal drip
PNF	proprioceptive neuromuscular facilitation
PNH	paroxysmal nocturnal hemoglobinuria
PNI	peripheral nerve injury • postnatal infection • psychoneuro- immunology
PNMT	phenylethanolamine N-methyltransferase
PNP	paranitrophenol • pediatric nurse practitioner • platelet neutralization procedure • psychogenic nocturnal polydipsia
PNPR	positive-negative pressure respiration
PNRS	premature nursery
PNS	parasympathetic nervous system • peripheral nervous system
PNT	percutaneous nephrostomy tube
Pnx	pneumothorax
po	by mouth *(per os)*
pO₂	partial pressure of oxygen

Po	ponomium
PO	parieto-occipital • phone order • postoperative • predominating organism
PO$_2$	partial pressure of oxygen
PO$_4$	phosphate
POA	pancreatic oncofetal antigen • primary optic atrophy
POB	penicillin in oil and beeswax • place of birth
POC	post-operative care • products of conception
pocul	cup *(poculum)*
POD	place of death • postoperative day • post-ovulatory day
Pod D	Doctor of Podiatry
PODx	pre-operative diagnosis
POF	pyruvate oxidation factor
pois	poison
polio	poliomyelitis
POLY	polymorphonuclear leukocyte
POMC	pro-opiomelanocortin
POMP	purinethol, Oncovin, methotrexate, prednisone
POMR	problem-oriented medical record
pop	popliteal (artery)
POP	2,5-diphenyloxazole • plasma osmotic pressure • Plaster of Paris • postoperative
POPOP	1,4-bis-(5-phenoxazole) benzene
POR	problem-oriented record
PORR	postoperative recovery room
pos	position • positive
POSC	problem-oriented system of charting
POSM	patient-operated selector mechanism
poss	possible

post	posterior • postmortem
POST	posterior
postgangl	postganglionic
post-op	postoperative
pot	potassium • potion
PotAGT	potential abnormality of glucose tolerance
poten	potential
POU	placenta, ovary, uterus
POW	prisoner of war
pp	polyphosphate • private patient
PP	near point of accommodation *(punctum proximum)* • partial pressure • pellagra preventive • Planned Parenthood • posterior pituitary • postpartum • postprandial • Preferred Provider • private patient • private practice • protoporphyrin • pulse pressure • pyrophosphate
P&P	prothrombin and proconvertin
ppa	after shaking the bottle *(phiala prius agitate)*
PPA	Planned Parenthood Association • Pittsburgh pneumonia agent • post-pill amenorrhea • preferred provider agreement • prudent purchase arrangement
ppb	parts per billion
PPB	positive-pressure breathing
PPBS	postprandial blood sugar
PPC	pooled platelet concentrate • progressive patient care
PPD	percussion and postural drainage • permanent partial disability • per patient day • postprandial • prepaid • purified protein derivative (tuberculin)
PPD-B	purified protein derivative - Battey
PPD-S	purified protein derivative - standard
PPE	partial plasma exchange • personal protective equipment

PPF	pellagra-preventive factor • phagocytosis-promoting factor • plasma protein fraction • purified protein fraction
ppg	picopicogram
PPG	photoplethysmograph, photoplethysmography • physician practice group
PPH	persistent pulmonary hypertension • postpartum hemorrhage • primary pulmonary hypertension
PPHx	previous psychiatric history
PPI	patient package insert • Plan Position Indication
Ppl	pleural pressure
PPLO	pleuropneumonia-like organism
ppm	parts per million • pulses per minute
PPM	permanent pacemaker
PPMM	postpolycythemia myeloid metaplasia
PPNG	penicillinase-producing *Neisseria gonorrhoeae*
PPO	pleuropneumonia organisms • preferred provider organization
PPP	pentose phosphate pathway • platelet-poor plasma
PPPPP	pain, pallor, pulse loss, paresthesia, paralysis
PPR	Price's precipitation reaction
PPS	post-partum sterilization • prospective payment system • prospective pricing system • protein plasma substitute
PPSH	pseudovaginal peritoneoscrotal hypospadias
ppt	precipitate
PPT	partial prothrombin time
pptd	precipitated
PPTL	post-partum tubal ligation
pptn	precipitation
PPVT	Peabody Picture Vocabulary Test

PQ	permeability quotient • Physician's Questionnaire
pr	pair • per rectum
Pr	praseodymium • presbyopia • prism
PR	far point of accommodation *(punctum remotum)* • partial remission • partial response • peer review • percentile rank • peripheral resistance • phenol red • physician reviewer • pityriasis rosea • pressoreceptor • proctologist • progesterone receptor • public relations • pulmonary rehabilitation • pulse rate
PRA	plasma renin activity
PRAC	practical • practice
PRAS	prereduced, anaerobically sterilized
PRBC	packed red blood cells
PRC	peer review committee • plasma renin concentration
PRD	paired domain • partial reaction of degeneration
PRE	physical reconditioning exercise • progressive resistive exercise
precip	precipitation
pref	preference
preg	pregnancy, pregnant
PREG	pregnenolone
pregn	pregnancy, pregnant
prelim	preliminary
pre-op	preoperative
prep	preparation, prepare
prev	prevention, preventive • previous
PrevAGT	previous abnormality of glucose tolerance
PRF	progressive renal failure • prolactin-releasing factor
PRFA	plasma-recognition-factor activity
PRH	prolactin-releasing hormone

primip	primipara
PRIST	paper radioimmunosorbent test
priv	private
PRK	photorefractive keratectomy
PRL	prolactin
prn	as needed *(pro re nata)*
PRN	pain resource nurse
pro	protein
Pro	proline
PRO	peer review organization • professional review organization • prolapse
prob	probable, probability • problem
proc	procedure
proct	proctology, proctologist
prod	produce, produced, product, production
PROEF	post-operative regimen for early oral feeding
prof	profession, professional • professor
prog	prognosis
PROG	progesterone
progn	prognosis
progr	progress
PROM	passive range of motion • premature rupture of membranes • prolonged rupture of membranes
PROPAC	Prospective Payment Assessment Commission
prostat	prostatic
proTime	prothrombin time
prox	proximal
prox luc	the day before *(proxima luce)*
PRP	platelet-rich plasma • polyribose ribitol phosphate • pressure-rate product

PRPP	phosphoribosylpyrophosphate
PRRB	Provider Reimbursement Review Board
PRT	phosphoribosyltransferase • photoradiation therapy
PRTase	phosphoribosyltransferase
PRU	peripheral resistance unit
PRVR	peak-to-resting-velocity ratio
ps	per second • picosecond
Ps	prescription • *Pseudomonas*
PS	chloropicrin • paradoxical sleep • paraseptal • pathologic stage • phosphatidylserine • physical status • plastic surgery • pregnancy serum • programmed symbols • pulmonary stenosis • pyloric stenosis
P/S	ratio of polyunsaturated to saturated fat
P&S	paracentesis and suction
PsA	psoriatic arthritis
PSA	prostate-specific antigen
PSAGN	poststreptococcal acute glomerulonephritis
PsAn	psychoanalysis, psychoanalyst
PSAP	prostate-specific acid phosphatase
PSBO	partial small bowel obstruction
PSC	posterior subcapsular cataract
PSD	peptone-starch-dextrose (agar) • posterior sagittal diameter
PSDA	Patient Self-Determination Act
PSE	partial systemic encephalopathy • point of subjective equality
PSG	pilot study group
PSH	postspinal headache
psi	pounds per square inch
PSI	personnel security index • posterior sagittal index

psia	pounds per square inch absolute
psig	pounds per square inch gauge
PSIS	posterior superior iliac spine
PSL	potassium, sodium chloride, sodium lactate (solution)
PSLT	Picture-Story Language Test
PSMA	progressive spinal muscular atrophy
PSP	phenolsulfonphthalein • progressive supra-nuclear palsy
PSR	problem status report
PSRBOW	premature spontaneous rupture of bag of waters
PSRO	professional standards review organization
PSS	physiologic saline solution • progressive systemic sclerosis (systemic scleroderma)
PST	pancreatic suppression test • paroxysmal supraventricular tachycardia • penicillin, streptomycin, tetracycline
PSVER	pattern-shift visual evoked response
PSVT	paroxysmal supraventricular tachycardia
PSW	psychiatric social worker
psy	psychiatry, psychology
psych	psychiatry, psychology
pt	part • patient • pint • point
Pt	platinum
PT	physical therapist, physical therapy • posterior tibial (pulse) • prothrombin time
PTA	percutaneous transluminal angioplasty • Physical Therapy Assistant • plasma thromboplastin antecedent • post-traumatic amnesia • prior to admission
PTAF	policy target adjustment factor
P-TAG	target-attaching globulin precursor

PTAP	purified diphtheria toxoid--alum precipitated
PTB	patellar tendon bearing • prior to birth
PTC	percutaneous transhepatic cholangiography • phenylthiocarbamide • plasma thromboplastin component • pseudotumor cerebri
PTCA	percutaneous transluminal coronary angioplasty
PTD	permanent and total disability
PTE	parathyroid extract • post-traumatic endophthalmitis • pretibial edema • pulmonary thromboembolism
PTF	plasma thromboplastin factor • post-transfusion fever
PTFE	polytetrafluoroethylene (graft, paste)
PTH	parathormone (parathyroid hormone) • phenylthiohydantoin • post-transfusion hepatitis
PTLD	post-transplant lymphoproliferative disease
PTN	provider telecommunication network
PTP	posterior tibial pulse
pts	patients
PTS	painful tonic seizure • permanent threshold shift • provider training sessions
PTSD	post-traumatic stress disorder
PTT	partial thromboplastin time
PTU	propylthiouracil
PTX	picrotoxin • pneumothorax
Pu	plutonium
PU	peptic ulcer • pregnancy urine
PuD	pulmonary disease
PUD	peptic ulcer disease
PUFA	polyunsaturated fatty acid
PUH	pregnancy urine hormone
pul	pulmonary

PULHES	physical profile: general Physical, Upper extremities, Lower extremities, Hearing, Eyes, pSychiatric
pulm	gruel *(pulmentum)* • pulmonary, pulmonic
pulv	powder *(pulvis)*
PUN	plasma urea nitrogen
PUO	pyrexia of undetermined origin • pyrexia of unknown origin
purg	purgative
PUVA	psoralen (oral) with long-wavelength ultraviolet light
PUVD	pulsed ultrasonic (blood) velocity detector
PUW	pick-up walker
PV	peripheral vascular • peripheral vein • plasma viscosity • plasma volume • polycythemia vera • portal vein • predictive value • pulmonary vein
PVA	polyvinyl alcohol
PVB	premature ventricular beat
PVC	polyvinyl chloride • post-voiding cystogram • premature ventricular contraction • pulmonary venous congestion
PVCO$_2$	mixed venous carbon dioxide pressure
PVD	peripheral vascular disease • premature ventricular depolarization
PVE	premature ventricular extrasystole
PVH	private voluntary hospital
PVM	pneumonia virus of mice
PVO$_2$	mixed venous oxygen pressure
PVOD	peripheral vascular occlusive disease
PVP	povidone (polyvinylpyrrolidone)
PVP-I	povidone (polyvinylpyrrolidone) iodine
PVR	peripheral vascular resistance • pulmonary vascular resistance • post-void residual

PVRI	peripheral vascular resistance index • pulmonary vascular resistance index
PVS	persistent vegetative state
PVSG	Polycythemia Vera Study Group
pvt	private
PVT	paroxysmal ventricular tachycardia • pressure, volume, temperature
P-W	Prader-Willi (syndrome)
PWA	person(s) with AIDS
PWB	partial weight-bearing
PWC	physical work capacity
PWLV	posterior wall of left ventricle
PWM	pokewood mitogen
PWOS	post-workout syncope
PWP	pulmonary wedge pressure
PWS	port-wine stain
Px	past history • pneumothorax • prognosis
PX	physical examination
PXE	pseudoxanthoma elasticum
Py	pyrene
PY	pack-year (cigarette use)
P/Y	pack-year (cigarete use)
pyr	pyridine
PZ	pancreozymin
PZA	pyrazinamide
PZI	protamine zinc insulin
PZP	pregnancy zone protein

Q

q	each, every *(quaque)* • four *(quattuor)* • quantity • quart • quartile • volume
Q	coulomb (electrical unit) • perfusion flow • quotient
Q°	perfusion (flow) rate
QA	quality assessment • quality assurance
QAC	Quality Assessment Committee • Quality Assessment Coordinator • Quality Assurance Committee • Quality Assurance Coordinator
QAD	Quality Assessment Director
qam	every morning
QAM	quality assurance monitoring
QAP	quality assurance program • quinine, atabrine, plasmoquine
QA / RM	quality assurance/risk management
QAT	quality action team
QA/UR	quality assurance/utilization review
QBCA	quantitative buffy-coat analysis
Q_C	pulmonary capillary blood flow (perfusion)
QC	quality control
QCIM	Quarterly Cumulative Index Medicus
Q_{CO_2}	number of microliters of CO_2 given off per mg. dry weight of tissue per hour
qd	every day *(quaque die)*
QEP	quality evaluation program
QES	quality education system
qh	every hour *(quaque hora)*

q2h	every two hours
q3h	every three hours
QI	quality improvement
qid	four times a day *(quater in die)*
QIP	quality improvement plan • quality improvement process • quality intervention plan
ql	as much as desired *(quantum libet)*
qm	every morning *(quaque mane)*
QM	quinacrine mustard
qn	every night *(quaque nocte)*
QNS	quantity not sufficient
QO$_2$	oxygen consumption • oxygen quotient
Q°O$_2$	oxygen consumption rate (microliters per milligram per hour)
qod	every other day
qoh	every other hour
qon	every other night
qp	at will, as much as desired *(quantum placeat)*
QP	quanti-Pirquet (reaction)
QPC	quality of patient care
qpm	every night
QP/QS	ratio of pulmonary to systemic circulation
qq	each *(quaque, quoque)*
qqh	every four hours *(quaque quarta hora)*
qq hor	every hour
QRN	quality review nurse
QRS	principal deflection in ECG
qs	quadriceps setting • quantity sufficient *(quantum satis)*
qt	quart • quiet

Qt	Quick's test
quad	quadrant • quadriceps • quadriplegia, quadriplegic
qual	qualitative • quality
qual anal	qualitative analysis
quant	quantitative
quant anal	quantitative analysis
quart	fourth *(quartus)*
quat	four *(quattuor)*
quats	quaternary ammonium compounds
quinq	five *(quinque)*
quint	fifth *(quintus)* • quintuplet
quot	daily *(quotidie)* • quotient
quotid	daily *(quotide)*
qv	as much as desired *(quantum vis)* • which see *(quod vide)*

R

r	far, remote *(remotum)* • rate • ring chromosome • roentgen
R	Behnken's unit (of roentgen-ray exposure) • organic radical • rad • radioactive • radiology, radiologist • range • Rankine (scale) • rate • Reaumur (scale) • rectal • red • reference • registered trademark • regression coefficient • resistance (electrical) • respiration • respiratory exchange ratio • response • reticulocyte • review • *Rickettsia* • right • Rinne's test (hearing) • roentgen
-R	Rinne's test negative
+R	Rinne's test positive
Ra	radium
RA	Radiation Oncology Services • Remittance Advice • renin activity • repeat action • residual air • rheumatoid arthritis • right angle • right arm • right atrial (pressure) • right atrium • right auricle • room air
RAA	renin-angiotensin-aldosterone (system) • right atrial abnormality
RA-ABG	room air arterial blood gases
rac	racemic
RAC	Recombinant DNA Advisory Committee • right atrial catheter
rad	radian • radiation absorbed dose • radical • radius • root *(radix)*
RAD	right anterior descending • right axis deviation
RADA	right acromio-dorso-anterior
RADCA	right anterior descending coronary artery

RADT	Radiation Therapy • registration, admission, discharge, transfer (system)
RAE	right atrial enlargement
RAEB	refractory anemia with excess of blasts
RAH	right anterior hemiblock • right atrial hypertrophy
RAHB	right anterior hemiblock
RAHTG	rabbit antihuman thymocyte globulin
RAI	radioactive iodine • right atrial involvement
RAIU	radioactive iodine uptake
RAM	random access memory
RAMC	Royal Army Medical Corps
RAMI	Risk Adjusted Mortality Index
RAN	resident's admission note
RANT	right anterior
RAO	right anterior oblique
RAP	Radiologists, Anesthesiologists, Pathologists • rheumatoid arthritis precipitin • right atrial pressure
RAR	right arm recumbent
ras	scrapings *(rasurae)*
RAS	regular analysts' sessions • reticular activating system
RAST	radioallergosorbent test • right anterior superior thorax
RAT	repeat action tablet • right anterior thorax
RAV	Rous-associated virus
RAW	airway resistance
Rb	rubidium
R&B	right and below
RBA	relative binding activity

RBB	right breast biopsy • right bundle branch
RBBB	right bundle branch block
RBBsB	right bundle branch system block
RBBX	right breast biopsy examination
RBC	red blood cell • red blood (cell) count
RBC-ADA	red-blood-cell adenosine deaminase
RBCD	right border of cardiac dullness
RBC frag	erythrocyte (red-blood-cell) fragility
RBD	regular blood donor • right-border dullness
RBE	relative biologic effectiveness
RBF	regional blood flow • renal blood flow
RBKA	right below-knee amputation
RBKLA	right below-knee leg amputation
RBOW	rupture of bag of waters
RBP	retinol-binding protein • right (arm) blood pressure
RC	radial-carpal • red cell • Red Cross • referred care • resource consumption • respirations ceased • respiratory center • right ear, cold stimulus
RCA	red-cell agglutination • Refugee Cash Assistance Program • right coronary artery
RCal	relative calories
rCBF	regional cerebral blood flow
RCC	ratio of costs to charges
RCCA	right common carotid artery
RCD	relative cardiac dullness
RCDR	relative corrected death rate
RCF	red-cell folate • relative centrifugal force
RCL	right coronary lesion
RCM	red-cell mass • right costal margin

RCP	resource consumption profile • Royal College of Physicians
RCPT	Registered Cardiopulmonary Technician
RCS	repeat cesarean section • reticulum-cell sarcoma • Royal College of Surgeons
RCT	random controlled trial • red cell toxin • Rorschach content test
RCU	red cell utilization • refined carbohydrate unit • renal care unit • respiratory care unit
RCV	red-cell volume
rd	rutherford (unit of radioactivity)
RD	Raynaud's disease • reaction of degeneration • registered dietitian • respiratory disease • retinal detachment • right deltoid • rubber dam
R&D	research and development
RdA	reading age
RDA	recommended dietary allowance • right dorsoanterior
RDC	Research Diagnostic Criteria
RDE	receptor-destroying enzyme
RDFS	ratio of decayed and filled surfaces (teeth)
RDFT	ratio of decayed and filled teeth
RDP	radiopharmaceutical drug product
RdQ	reading quotient
RDRC	Radioactive Drug Research Committee
RDS	respiratory distress syndrome • reticuloendothelial depressing substance
RDT	regular dialysis treatment
RDW	red (cell) distribution width
re	concerning
Re	rhenium

RE	radium emanation • regional enteritis • reticuloendothelial • retinol equivalent • right extremity • right eye
react	reaction
readm	readmission
rec	fresh *(recens)* • recommendation • record • recreation • recurrent
REC	radioelectrocomplexing
RECA	right external carotid artery
Rec Asst	recreation assistant
RECG	radioelectrocardiography
recip	recipient • reciprocal
recond	recondition
reconstr	reconstruction
recryst	recrystallize
Rec Spec	recreation specialist
rect	rectal • rectified
Rec Tech	recreation technician
red	reduce, reducing, reduction
redn	reduction
REEGT	Registered Electroencephalographic Technician
REEP	role exchange/education practice
ref	refer, referred • reference
REF	renal erythropoietic factor
ref doc	referring doctor
refl	reflex
reg	region • regular
Reg	registered
REG	radioencephalogram
regen	regenerate, regeneration

reg umb	umbilical region
regurg	regurgitate
rehab	rehabilitation
rel	related, relative
REL	rate of energy loss
rem	roentgen equivalent man (unit of radiation exposure)
REM	rapid-eye-movement (sleep)
rep	let it be repeated *(repetatur)* • roentgen equivalent physical
REP	repeat • report
rept	repeat • report
req	required
res	research • reserve • residence • resident • residue
RES	electrical resistance • reticuloendothelial system
resc	resuscitation
resp	respective, respectively • respiration, respiratory • responsible
ret	retired
retic	reticulocyte
rev	reverse • review • revolutions
rev/min	revolutions per minute
rf	radiofrequency
Rf	retardation factor
RF	Reitland-Franklin (unit) • relative flow (rate) • releasing factor • rheumatic fever • rheumatoid factor
RFA	right femoral artery • right forearm • right frontoanterior
RFFIT	rapid fluorescent focus inhibition test
RFL	right frontolateral

RFLP	restriction fragment length polymorphism
RFP	right frontoposterior
RFR	refraction
RFT	right frontotransverse
RG	right gluteal, right gluteus
RGE	relative gas expansion
Rh	rhesus (blood factor) • rhodium • rhonchi
RH	radiant heat • Rehabilitation Services • relative humidity • releasing hormone • right hand
RHC	regional heart center • respirations have ceased
RHD	relative hepatic dullness • rheumatic heart disease • rural healthcare delivery
rheum	rheumatic
RHF	right heart failure
RHG	relative hemoglobin
RHH	right homonymous hemianopsia
Rhig	Rh immunoglobulin
rhin	rhinology, rhinologist • rhinorrhea
rhm	roentgens per hour at one meter
RHP	regional health planning • right hemiparesis • right hemiplegia
RHV	right hepatic vein
RI	input resistors • refractive index • respiratory illness • retroactive inhibition
RIA	radioimmunoassay
RIA-DA	radioimmunoassay - double antibody
Rib	ribose
RIC	right iliac crest • right internal capsule • right internal carotid
RICA	right internal carotid artery

RICE	rest, ice, compression, elevation
RICM	right intercostal margin
RICS	right intercostal space
RICU	respiratory intensive-care unit
RID	radial immunodiffusion
RIF	rifampin • right iliac fossa
RIG	rabies immune globulin
RIH	right inguinal hernia
RIHSA	radioiodinated human serum albumin
RIMA	right internal mammary artery
RIND	reversible ischemic neurologic deficit
RIPA	radioimmunoprecipitation assay
RISA	radioiodinated serum albumin
RIST	radioimmunosorbent test
RIVS	ruptured interventricular septum
RK	radial keratotomy • right kidney
RKY	roentgen kymography
rl	fine rales
Rl	medium rales
RL	coarse rales • right lateral • right leg • right lower • right lung • Ringer's lactate
R-L	right to left
R/L	right to left
R Lat	right lateral
R LAT	right lateral
RLBCD	right lower border of cardiac dullness
RLC	residual lung capacity
RLD	related living donor • right lateral decubitus (position) • ruptured lumbar disc

RLE	right lower extremity
RLF	retrolental fibroplasia • right lateral femoral
rll	right lower lid
RLL	right lower lobe
RLQ	right lower quadrant
RLR	right lateral rectus
RLSB	right lower sternal border
RLT	right lateral thigh
RLV	Rauscher leukemia virus
RM	radical mastectomy • range of motion • respiratory movement • risk management
RMA	right mentoanterior
RMB	right main-stem bronchus
RMCA	right main coronary artery
RMCL	right midclavicular line
RMD	retromanubrial dullness
RMK	rhesus monkey kidney
RML	right mediolateral • right middle lobe
RMLS	right middle lobe syndrome
RMP	regional medical program • resting membrane potential • right mentoposterior
RMPS	regional medical program service
RMR	resting metabolic rate • right medial rectus
RMS	square root of mean square
RMSF	Rocky Mountain spotted fever
RMT	right mentotransverse
RMV	respiratory minute volume
Rn	radon
RN	registered nurse • renal disease

RNA	ribonucleic acid
RNase	ribonuclease
RN,C	Registered Nurse, Certified
RN,CNAA	Registered Nurse, Certified in Nursing Administrated, Advanced
RN,CS	Registered Nurse, Certified Specialist
RNICU	regional neonatal intensive-care unit
RNIP	Registered Nurse, Interim Permit
RNMS	registered nurse of the mentally subnormal
RNP	registered nurse-practitioner • ribonucleoprotein
RNS	reference normal serum
Rnt	roentgenology, roentgenologist
RNV	radionuclide venography
RO	routine order
R/O	rule out
ROA	right occipitoanterior
ROC	receiver operating characteristic
ROE	return on equity
ROL	right occipitolateral
ROM	range of motion • read-only memory • rupture of membranes
ROP	retinopathy of prematurity • right occipitoposterior
ROS	Radiation Oncology Services • review of systems
rot	rotate, rotated, rotation, rotating
ROT	remedial occupational therapy • right occipitotransverse
ROW	Rendu-Osler-Weber syndrome
RP	radial pulse • Raynaud's phenomenon • refractory period • Respiratory Care Services • retinitis pigmentosa

RPA	right pulmonary artery
RPCF	Reiter protein complement fixation (test)
RPF	relaxed pelvic floor • renal plasma flow
RPG	radiation protection guide
RPGN	rapidly progressive glomerulonephritis
RPHA	reverse passive hemagglutination
RPI	reticulocyte production index
RPICA	right posterior internal carotid artery
RPLND	retroperitoneal lymph node dissection
rpm	revolutions per minute
RPO	right posterior oblique
R POST	right posterior
RPP	retropubic prostatectomy
RPR	rapid plasma reagin (test)
rps	revolutions per second
RPS	renal pressor substance • review per screen
rpt	repeat • report
RPT	registered physical therapist • right posterior thorax
RPV	right portal vein
RQ	recovery quotient • respiratory quotient
RR	radiation response • recovery room • regular respirations • relative risk • respiratory rate
R&R	rate and rhythm • rest and relaxation
RRA	radioreceptor assay • Registered Record Administrator
RRC	recruitment and retention committee
RRE	radiation-related eosinophilia
RR&E	round, regular, and equal (pupils)
rRNA	ribosomal ribonucleic acid

RRP	Refugee Resettlement Program • relative refractory period
RRR	regular rate and rhythm (heart)
RRRN	round, regular, react normally
RRT	registered respiratory therapist
RRV	rhesus rotavirus vaccine
RRx	radiation prescription
Rs	respond, response
RS	*Rauwolfia serpentina* • reinforcing stimulus • Reiter's syndrome • respiratory system • review of systems • Reye's syndrome • Ringer's solution
R-S	reticulated siderocytes
RSA	right sacroanterior • right subclavian artery
RSB	right sternal border
RScA	right scapuloanterior
RScP	right scapuloposterior
RSD	reflex sympathetic dystrophy • relative standard deviation
R-SICU	respiratory-surgical intensive-care unit
RSIVP	rapid sequence intravenous pyelogram
RSNA	Radiological Society of North America
RSO	radiation safety officer • right salpingo-oophorectomy
RSP	right sacroposterior
RSR	regular sinus rhythm
RSSE	Russian spring-summer encephalitis
RST	radiosensitivity test • rapid surfactant test • reagin screen test • right sacrotransverse
RSV	Rous sarcoma virus
RSW	right-sided weakness
rt	right

RT	radiologic technician, technologist • radiotherapy • radium therapy • reaction time • reading time • reciprocating tachycardia • recreational therapy, therapist • registered technician, technologist • respiratory therapy, therapist • right triceps • room temperature
RTA	renal tubular acidosis
RTC	residential treatment center • return to clinic
RTD	resubmission turnaround documents
RTech	radiology technologist, technician
RTF	residential treatment facility • resistance transfer factor • respiratory tract fluid
rtn	return
RTN	Registered Technologist, Nuclear Medicine • routine
RTO	return to office
RTR	Registered Technologist, Radiography
RTT	Radiation Therapy Technician
RT$_3$U	resin T$_3$ (triiodothyronine) uptake (test)
RTUS	real time ultrasonography
Ru	ruthenium
RU	radioulnar • rat unit • rectourethral • residual urine • retrograde urogram • roentgen unit
RUA	right upper arm
rub	red *(ruber)*
RUE	right upper extremity
RUG	Resource Utilization Group
rul	right upper lid
RUL	right upper leg • right upper lobe
RUO	right ureteral orifice
rupt	rupture
RUQ	right upper quadrant

RURTI	recurrent upper respiratory tract infection
RV	residual volume • retroversion • right ventricle, ventricular • rubella vaccine
RVA	right ventricular abnormality
RVD	relative vertebral density • rest vertical dimension • right ventricular dimension
RVDO	right ventricular diastolic overload
RVE	right ventricular enlargement
RVEDP	right ventricular end-diastolic pressure
RVEDV	right ventricular end-diastolic volume
RVET	right ventricular ejection time
RVFP	right ventricular filling pressure
RVG	radionuclide ventriculogram, ventriculography
RVH	renovascular hypertension • right ventricular hypertrophy
RVID	right ventricular internal dimension
RVIDP	right ventricular initial diastolic pressure
RVLG	right ventrolateral gluteal
RVO	relaxed vaginal outlet • right ventricular outflow • right ventricular overactivity
RVP	right ventricular pressure
RVR	renal vein renin
RVS	Relative Value Scale • Relative Value Schedule • Relative Value Studies
RVSW	right ventricular stroke work
RVSWI	right ventricular stroke work index
RVV	rubella vaccine virus
RW	right ear, warm stimulus
Rx	prescription • take *(recipe)* • treatment

S

s̄	without *(sine)* • without spectacles
S	half *(semis)* • left *(sinister)* • mark *(signa)* • sacral (nerve, vertebra) • saline • saturation • second • section • sedimentation coefficient • sensation • sensitive • serum • siderocyte • single • smooth (bacterial colony) • soft (diet) • soluble • son • spherical (lens) • stimulus • subject • sulfur • supravergence • surgery, surgical, surgeon • Svedberg unit
S1-S5	sacral vertebrae 1 through 5
SA	salicylic acid • short-acting • sialoadenectomy • sinoatrial • specific activity • Stokes-Adams (disease) • suicide awareness • surface area • surgeon's assistant • sustained-action
S/A	sugar and acetone
SAARD	slow-acting antirheumatic drug
SAB	Society of American Bacteriologists • spontaneous abortion
SAC	short arm cast
sacc	cogwheel (respiration)
SACD	subacute combined degeneration
SACE	serum angiotensin-converting enzyme
SACH	solid ankle, cushion heel (foot prosthesis)
SACT	sinoatrial conduction time
SAD	seasonal affective disorder • Self-Assessment Depression Scale • sugar, acetone, diacetic acid (test)
SADBE	squaric acid dibutylester
SADS	Schedule for Affective Disorders and Schizophrenia

SAECG	signal-averaged electrocardiogram
SAED	selected area electron diffraction
SAFA	soluble-antigen fluorescent antibody (test)
SAFE	stationary attachment, flexible endoskeleton (foot prosthesis)
SAH	subarachnoid hemorrhage
SAID	sexually acquired immunodeficiency syndrome • steroidal anti-inflammatory drugs
Sal	*Salmonella*
SAM	self-administered medication • systolic anterior motion
SAN	sinoatrial node
sanit	sanitarium • sanitary, sanitation
SAO	Southeast Asian Ovalocytosis
SAO$_2$	arterial blood oxygen saturation
sap	saponify, saponification
SAP	serum alkaline phosphate
SAPD	self-administration of psychotropic drugs
SAPMS	short arm posterior molded splint
sapon	saponify, saponification
SAQ	short-arc quadriceps test
SART	sinoatrial recovery time
SAS	space-adaptation syndrome • sterile aqueous suspension • subarachnoid space
sat	saturate, saturated
SAT	Scholastic Aptitude Test
satis	satisfactory
SATL	surgical Achilles tendon lengthening
Sb	antimony *(stibium)* • strabismus

SB	Sengstaken-Blakemore (tube) • sideroblas... bradycardia • small bowel • spina bifid... Stanford-Binet (test) • stillbirth, stillborn suction biopsy
+SB	wearing seat belts
SBA	stand-by assistance
SBB	specialist in blood bank
SBE	shortness of breath on exertion • subacute bacterial endocarditis
SBFT	small bowel follow-through
SBGM	self blood-glucose monitoring
SBJ	skin, bones, joints
SBMPL	simultaneous binaural midplace localization
SBN$_2$	single-breath nitrogen (test)
SBO	small bowel obstruction
SBOD	scleral buckle, right eye
SBOS	scleral buckle, left eye
SBP	spontaneous bacterial peritonitis • systolic blood pressure
SBR	strict bed rest
SBS	small bowel series • staff burn-out scale
SBTI	soybean trypsin inhibitor
SBSM	self blood sugar monitoring
Sc	scandium
SC	sacrococcygeal • secretory coil • self care • semilunar (valves) closure • service-connected • sickle cell • stimulus, conditioned • subcorneal • subcutaneous • sugar-coated • supportive care
S/C	supraclavicular
SCAN	suspected child abuse and neglect
SCAT	sheep-cell agglutination test • sickle-cell anemia test

ꜱCB	strictly confined to bed
SCC	squamous cell carcinoma
ScD	Doctor of Science
SCD	service-connected disability • sudden cardiac death
ScDA	right scapuloanterior *(scapulodextra anterior)*
ScDP	right scapuloposterior *(scapulodextra posterior)*
SCE	sister-chromatid exchange
SCG	sodium cromoglycate
SCH	sole community hospital
sched	schedule
SCHNC	squamous cell head and neck cancer
sci	science • scientific
SCI	spinal cord injury
SCIU	spinal cord injury unit
SCID	severe combined immunodeficiency disease
SCIPP	sacrococcygeal to inferior pubic point
SCL	scleroderma • serum copper level • soft contact lens
ScLA	left scapuloanterior *(scapulolaeva anterior)*
SCLC	small-cell lung carcinoma
ScLP	left scapuloposterior *(scapulolaeva posterior)*
SCM	state-certified midwife • sternocleidomastoid muscle
SCN	self-care needs
SCO	supportive care only
scop	scopolamine
SCP	single-celled protein
SCPK	serum creatine phosphokinase
Scr	scruple • serum creatinine
SCR	spondylitic caudal radiculopathy

SCRAP	Simple Complex Reaction-Time Apparatus
SCT	salmon calcitonin • sentence-completion test • sickle-cell trait • staphylococcal clumping test • sugar-coated tablet
SCU	Special Care Unit
SCUBA	self-contained underwater breathing apparatus
SCV	smooth, capsulated, virulent (bacteria)
SD	senile dementia • septal defect • serologically defined (antigen) • skin dose • spontaneous delivery • standard deviation • sterile dressing • straight drainage • streptodornase • sudden death
SDA	right sacroanterior (*sacrodextra anterior*) • specific dynamic action • succinate dehydrogenase activity
SDAT	senile dementia of the Alzheimer's type
SDE	specific dynamic effect
SDH	sorbitol dehydrogenase • subdural hematoma • succinate dehydrogenase
SDL	self-directed learning
SDLRS	self-directed-learning readiness scale
SDM	standard deviation of the mean
SDP	right sacroposterior (*sacrodextra posterior*) • single-donor platelets
SDS	same-day surgery
SDT	right sacrotransverse (*sacrodextra transversa*)
Se	selenium
SE	saline enema • *Salmonella enteridities* • spherical equivalent • spin echo • standard error (of the mean)
S-E	Starr-Edwards (prosthesis)
SEA	sheep erythrocyte agglutination (test) • Southeast Asia • spontaneous electrical activity
SEAL	Southeast Asian learners
SEAR	Southeast Asian refugees

sec	second • secondary
SEC	soft elastic capsules • squamous epithelial cells
sect	section
sed	stool *(sedes)*
SED	skin erythema dose
SEER	surveillance, epidemiology and end results
sed rate	(erythrocyte) sedimentation rate
seg	segment, segmented • segmented cell
SEG	sonoencephalogram, sonoencephalography
sem	semen
SEM	scanning electron microscope • standard error of the mean • systolic ejection murmur
semih	half an hour *(semihora)*
SENA	sympathetic efferent nerve activity
SENIC	Study on the Efficacy of Nosocomial Infection Control
sens	sensitivity
SENTAC	Society for Ear, Nose and Throat Advances in Children
SEO	surgical emergency officer
sep	separately
SEP	sensory evoked potential • somatosensory evoked potential • systolic ejection period
seq	that which follows *(sequela)*
seq luce	the following day *(sequenti luce)*
ser	series • service
Ser	serine
SER	somatosensory evoked response • systolic ejection rate
sero	serology

serv	keep *(serva)* • preserve
SES	socioeconomic status
SET	skin endpoint titration
sev	severe • severed
SeXO	serum xanthine oxidase
S$_f$	Svedberg flotation unit
SF	salt-free • scarlet fever • slow initial function • spinal fluid • stress formula • synovial fluid
SFA	serum folate • superficial femoral angioplasty
SFC	spinal fluid count
SFD	skin-to-film distance • small-for-dates
SFEMG	single-fiber electromyography
SFP	screen-filtration pressure • spinal-fluid pressure
SFR	screen-filtration resistance
SG	signs • skin graft • soluble gelatin • specific gravity • Surgeon-General • surgery • survey group • Swan-Ganz (catheter)
S-G	Sachs-Georgi (test)
SGA	small for gestational age
SGAW	specific airway conductance
SGE	significant glandular enlargement
SGF	skeletal growth factor
SGGT	serum gamma-glutamyltransferase
SGO	Surgeon General's Office
SGOT	serum glutamic-oxaloacetic transaminase
SGPT	serum glutamic-pyruvic transaminase
sh	shoulder
Sh	*Shigella* • short
SH	serum hepatitis • social history • somatotropic hormone • sulfhydryl • surgical history

SHARE	Siblings Helping Persons with Autism through Resources and Energy
SHBD	serum hydroxybutyrate dehydrogenase
SHCC	Statewide Health Coordinating Council
SHHH	Self Help for Hard of Hearing People
shld	shoulder
SHP	Schonlein-Henoch purpura
SHPDA	State Health Planning and Development Agency
SHSWD	Society for Hospital Social Work Directors
Si	silicon
SI	sacroiliac • saturation index • seriously ill • serum iron • soluble insulin • special intervention • stroke index • *Systeme International d'Unites*
SIADH	syndrome of inappropriate secretion of antidiuretic hormone
sib	sibling
SICU	surgical intensive-care unit
SID	Society for Investigative Dermatology
SIDS	sudden infant death syndrome
SIE	stroke in evolution • subacute infective endocarditis
SIECUS	Sex Information and Education Council of the United States
sig	let it be labeled *(signetur)* • signal • significant
SIg	surface immunoglobulin
SIG	sigmoidoscope, sigmoidoscopy
sig n pro	label with the proper name *(signa nomine proprio)*
SI/IS	severity of illness/intensity of services
SIJ	sacroiliac joint
SIMS	surgical indication monitoring system
simul	simultaneously

SIMV	synchronous intermittent mandatory ventilation
sin	without *(sine)*
sing	of each *(singulorum)*
si op sit	if it is necessary *(si opus sit)*
SIP	sickness impact profile
SISI	short (small)-increment sensitivity index
SIW	self-inflicted wound
S-J	Stevens-Johnson syndrome
SK	streptokinase
SKIP	Sick Kids need Involved People
SKSD	streptokinase-streptodornase
sl	slight
SL	sensation level • slit lamp • staphage lysate • sublingual
SLA	left sacroanterior *(sacrolaeva anterior)* • slide latex agglutination
SLB	short leg brace
SLC	short leg cast
SLE	St. Louis encephalitis • systemic lupus erythematosus
SLFIA	substrate-labeled fluorescent immunoassay • substrate-linked fluorescent immunoassay
SLM	spatial light modulator
SLO	streptolysin-O
SLP	left sacroposterior *(sacrolaeva posterior)*
SLPMS	short leg posterior molded splint
SLR	straight-leg-raising (test)
SLT	left sacrotransverse *(sacrolaeva transversa)*
SLWC	short leg walking cast
sm	small

Sm	samarium • symptoms
SM	smooth muscle • streptomycin • systolic murmur
SMA	schedule of maximum allowance • Sequential Multiple Analyzer • smooth muscle antibody • spinal muscular atrophy • superior mesenteric artery
SMAC	Sequential Multiple Analyzer with Computer
SMBG	self-monitored blood glucose
SMD	senile macular degeneration • submanubrial dullness
sm-FeSV	McDonough feline sarcoma virus
SMH	state mental hospital
SMI	Supplementary (Medicare) Insurance Program
SMO	school medical office, officer • senior medical officer
SMON	subacute myelo-opticoneuropathy
SMR	somnolent metabolic rate • Standardized Mortality Rate, Ratio • submucous resection
SMT	stress management training • student medical technologist
SMX	sulfamethoxazole
SMZ	sulfamethoxazole
Sn	tin *(stannum)*
SN	according to nature *(secundum naturam)* • school of nursing • serum neutralization, serum neutralizing • staff nurse • student nurse
S/N	sample-to-negative control ratio • signal-to-noise ratio
SNA	Student Nurses' Association • systems network architecture
SNAB	Staff Nurse Advisory Board
SNCV	sensory-nerve conduction velocity
SNDO	Standard Nomenclature of Diseases and Operations

SNE	subacute necrotizing encephalomyopathy
SNEC	Staff Nurse Executive Committee
SNF	skilled nursing facility
SNF/MR	skilled nursing facility for the mentally retarded
SNGFR	single-nephron glomerular filtration rate
SNM	Society of Nuclear Medicine
SNO	substantive negative outcome
SNOMED	Standardized Nomenclature of Medicine
SNOP	Standard Nomenclature of Pathology
SNS	Society of Neurological Surgeons • sympathetic nervous system
SO	salpingo-oophorectomy • significant other • Social Work Services • suicidal observation • superior oblique • supraoptic
sO$_2$	blood oxygen saturation
SO$_2$	blood oxygen saturation
SOAP	Subjective, Objective, Assessment, Plan (problem-oriented record)
SOAPS	suction, oxygen, apparatus, pharmaceuticals, saline
SOB	shortness of breath • suboccipitobregmatic
soc	social • society
SOC	standard of care
SOI	severity of illness
sol	soluble • solution
SOL	space-occupying lesion
soln	solution
solu	solute
solv	dissolve *(solve)* • solvent
SOM	serous otitis media
SONP	soft organs not palpable

SOP	standard operating procedure
s op s	if necessary *(si opus sit)*
S-O-R	stimulus-organism-response
sos	if necessary *(si opus sit)*
SOTT	synthetic-medium old tuberculin, trichloroacetic acid-precipitated
SOW	scope of work
sp	space • species • specific • spine, spinal • spirit (alcohol)
s/p	status post
Sp	sacropubic
SP	special care services • sulfapyridine • suprapubic • systolic pressure
SPA	salt-poor albumin • spondyloarthropathy
span.	spansule
SPBI	serum protein-bound iodine
SPBT	suprapubic bladder tap
SPCA	serum prothrombin conversion accelerator
SPD	salmon-poisoning disease • sterile processing department
SPDT	single-pole double-throw (switch)
SPE	serum protein electrophoresis
spec	specimen
SPEP	serum protein electrophoresis
SPF	specific pathogen-free • sun protection (protective) factor
SPFC	suprapubic Foley catheter
sp fl	spinal fluid
SPG	specific gravity • sucrose-phospate-glutamate
sp gr	specific gravity

sph	spherical • spherical lens
SPI	serum-precipitable iodine
spkr	speaker
SPMA	spinal progressive muscular atrophy
SPN	student practical nurse
spon	spontaneous
spont	spontaneous
spp	species
SPP	suprapubic prostatectomy
SPPS	stable plasma-protein solution
SPS	systemic progressive sclerosis
SPST	single-pole, single-throw (switch)
SPT	skin prick test
SPU	short procedure unit
SPV	slow-phase velocity
sq	square
SQ	subcutaneous
SQC	semiquantitative culture
SqCCA	squamous-cell carcinoma
SqCCAL	squamous-cell carcinoma of the lung
sq cm	square centimeter
sq ft	square foot
SQUID	Superconducting Quantum Interference Devices
sq m	square meter
sq mm	square millimeter
Sr	strontium

SR	sarcoplasmic reticulum • saturation-recovery • secretion rate • sedimentation rate • senior • sensitization response • sex ratio • side rails • sinus rhythm • stimulus-response • stomach rumble • sustained release • systems review
SRAW	specific airway resistance
SRBC	sheep red blood cells
SRBOW	spontaneous rupture of bag of waters
SRE	Schedule of Recent Experience
SRF	skin reactive factor • slow-reacting factor • somatotropin-releasing factor
SRF-A	slow-reacting factor of anaphylaxis
SRFC	sheep red-cell rosette-forming cells
SRH	single radial hemolysis • spontaneously resolving hyperthyroidism • stigmata of recent hemorrhage
SRIF	somatotropin release-inhibiting factor
SRMC	single room maternity care
sRNA	soluble ribonucleic acid
SR/NE	sinus rhythm, no ectopy
SROM	spontaneous rupture of membranes
SRR	surgical recovery room
SRRS	Social Readjustment Rating Scale
SRS	slow-reacting substance • Social Rehabilitation Service
SRS-A	slow-reacting substance of anaphylaxis
SRT	sedimentation rate test • speech reception threshold
SRU	side rails up
ss	one-half *(semis)*

SS	saline soak • saliva sample • saturated solution • sea sickness • serum sickness • Sézary syndrome • siblings • side to side • single -stranded (DNA) • soapsuds • social services • standard score • sterile solution • steroid sulfurylation • suction socket • sulfasalazine
S/S	signs and symptoms
SSA	*Salmonella-Shigella* agent • skin-sensitizing antibody • Social Security Administration
SSD	source-to-skin distance
SSDI	Social Security Disability Income
SSE	soapsuds enema
SSEP	somato-sensory evoked potential
SSI	segmental sequential irradiation • Supplemental Security Income
SSKI	saturated solution of potassium iodide
SSM	superficial spreading melanoma
SSOP	Second Surgical Opinion Program
SSPE	subacute sclerosing panencephalitis
SSR	surgical supply room
SSRI	selective serotonin re-uptake inhibitor
SSPL	saturation sound pressure level
sss	layer upon layer *(stratum super stratum)*
SSS	sick sinus syndrome • specific soluble substance • sterile saline soak • strong soap solution
SSSS	staphylococcal scalded-skin syndrome
SSSV	superior sagittal sinus-blood velocity
SSU	Saybolt seconds universal
ssv	under a poison label *(sub signo veneni)*
SSV	simian sarcoma virus
st	let it stand *(stet)* • straight

St	subtype
ST	sedimentation time • serum transferrin • sinus tachycardia • skin test • slight trace • standardized test • sublingual tablet • surface tension • surgical technologist • survival time
STA	serum thrombotic accelerator
staph	staphylococcus, staphylococcal
stat	immediately *(statim)*
stb	stillborn
STB	silicotuberculosis
STC	stroke treatment center
std	standard
STD	sexually transmitted disease • short-term disability • skin-test dose • sodium tetradecyl sulfate • standard test dose
STET	submaximal treadmill exercise test
STF	specialized treatment facility
ST-FeSv	Snyder-Thielen feline sarcoma virus
STH	somatotropic hormone
S-Thal	hemoglobin S and thalassemia
stim	stimulation
STK	streptokinase
STM	short-term memory • streptomycin
STP	dimethoxymethylamphetamine (hallucinogenic drug) • standard temperature and pressure
STPD	standard temperature and pressure-dry
str	*Streptococcus*
strep	*Streptococcus*
struct	structure

STS	serologic test for syphilis • Society of Thoracic Surgeons • standard test for syphilis • sugar-tong splint
STSG	split-thickness skin graft
STU	skin-test unit
su	let him take *(sumat)*
SU	sensation unit • strontium unit
S&U	supine and upright
SUA	serum uric acid
subcu	subcutaneous
subq	subcutaneous
subst	substance
SUD	skin unit dose • sudden unexpected death
SUDS	single-unit delivery system • sudden unexpected death syndrome
SUID	sudden unexplained infant death
sum	let him take *(sumat)* • summation
SUN	serum urea nitrogen
sup	superficial • superior • supervision, supervisor
supp	support • suppository
surg	surgeon, surgery, surgical
susp	suspension
sv	alcoholic spirit *(spiritus vini)* • single vibration
SV	simian virus • sinus venosus • spoken voice • spontaneous ventilation • stroke volume
SV4O	simian vacuolating virus 40
SVC	slow vital capacity • superior vena cava • suprahepatic vena cava
SVCS	superior vena cava syndrome
SVE	sterile vaginal examination • supraventricular ectopy

SVG	saphenous-vein graft
SVI	stroke volume index
SVPB	supraventricular premature beat
SVR	systemic vascular resistance
SVRI	systemic vascular resistance index
SVT	supraventricular tachycardia
sw	switch
SW	social worker
SWB	salaries, wages, benefits
SWD	short-wave diathermy
SWI	stroke work index • surgical wound infection
SWR	serum Wassermann reaction
SWS	slow-wave sleep
Sx	signs • symptoms
sym	symmetrical
symp	symptoms
syn	syndrome
sync	synchronous
synch	synchronous
synth	synthetic
Syph	syphilis
syr	syringe • syrup
sys	system, systemic
syst	systemic • systolic
Sz	seizure

T

t	life (time) • temporal • three times (ter) • ton (metric) • translocation (in genetics)
T	life (time) • obtained under test conditions • temperature • tension (pressure) • tera- • tesla (unit of magnetic flux density) • thoracic (nerve, vertebra) • thymine • tidal (volume) • tocopherol • tonometer reading • topical (medication) • total • transition point • transverse • *Treponema* • tritium
T-	decreased tension (pressure)
T+	increased tension (pressure)
t1/2	half-life (time)
T1/2	half-life (time)
T$_1$	monoiodotyrosine
T$_2$	diiodotyrosine
T$_3$	triiodothyronine
T$_4$	tetraiodothyronine (thyroxine)
T1-T12	thoracic vertebra 1 through 12
Ta	tantalum
TA	temperature, axillary • thyroglobulin autoprecipitation • toxin-antitoxin • transactional analysis • transaldolase • transantral • tryptophan-acid (reaction)
T&A	tonsillectomy and adenoidectomy
TAA	tumor-associated antigen
tab	tablet
TAB	therapeutic abortion • typhoid, paratyphoid A, paratyphoid B

TACE	chlorotrianisene (trianisylchloroethylene)
tachy	tachycardia
TAD	transverse abdominal diameter
TAF	tissue angiogenesis factor • tumor angiogenesis factor
TAG	target-attaching globulin
TAH	total abdominal hysterectomy • total artificial heart
tal	such (*talis*)
TAM	toxin-antitoxin mixture • toxoid-antitoxoid mixture • treat arrhythmias medically
TAME	tosyl-*L*-arginine methyl ester
tan	tangent
TANI	total axial (lymph) node irradiation
TAO	thromboangiitis obliterans • troleandomycin (triacetyloleandomycin)
TAPVC	total anomalous pulmonary venous connection
TAPVD	total anomalous pulmonary venous drainage
TAQW	transient abnormal Q waves
TAR	thrombocytopenia-absent radius (syndrome) • treatment authorization request
TARA	tumor-associated rejection antigen
TAT	tetanus antitoxin • Thematic Apperception Test • toxin-antitoxin • turnaround time • tyrosine aminotransferase
t$_b$	biologic half-life
Tb	terbium • tubercle bacillus
TB	thymol blue • toluidine blue • total body • tuberculosis
TBA	tertiary butylacetate • thiobarbituric acid • to be admitted • tumor-bearing animal
TBC	tuberculosis, tuberculous

TBG	testosterone-binding globulin • thyroxine-binding globulin
TBI	total-body irradiation
TBII	TSH-binding inhibitory immunoglobulin
TBIL	total bilirubin
TBili	total bilirubin
TBLC	term birth, live child
TBM	tuberculous meningitis
TBNA	total-body neutron activation
TBP	bithionol (thiobisdichlorophenol) • thyroxine-binding protein
TBR	total bed rest
TBS	tribromsalan (tribromosalicylanilide)
TBSA	total burn surface area
tbsp	tablespoonful
Tb-T	tracheobronchial toilet
TBT	transcervical balloon tuboplasty
TBV	total blood volume
TBW	total body water
Tc	technetium
^{99m}Tc	technetium metastable radionuclide used in diagnostic scanning
TC	tetracycline • therapeutic concentrate • throat culture • tissue culture • to contain • transplant center • treatment completed • tuberculosis, contagious • tubocurarine
T&C	turn and cough • type and crossmatch
TCA	tricarboxylic acid • trichloroacetate • trichloroacetic acid • tricyclic amine • tricyclic antidepressant
TCAP	trimethylcetylammonium pentachlorophenate

TCB	to call back
TCBS	thiosulfate-citrate-bile salts-sucrose (agar)
TCC	transitional cell carcinoma
TCD	tissue culture dose
TCD$_{50}$	median tissue culture dose
TCDB	turn, cough, deep breath
TCE	trichloroethylene
T-cells	thymus-dependent cells (lymphocytes)
TCGF	T-cell growth factor
TCI	tricuspid insufficiency
TCID	tissue culture infective dose
TCID$_{50}$	median tissue culture infective dose
TCM	tissue culture medium
TCMI	T-cell-mediated immunity
TCN	transcultural nursing
TcPO$_2$	transcutaneous PO$_2$ monitor
TCT	thrombin clotting time
TD	tardive dyskinesia • thoracic duct • time disintegration • to deliver • torsion dystonia • total disability • transverse diameter • tumor dose • typhoid dysentery
T$_4$D	thyroxine displacement (assay)
TDA	therapeutic drug assay • thyroid-stimulating hormone-displacing antibody • tryptophan deaminase agar
TDD	thoracic-duct drainage • total digitalizing dose
TDI	toluene diisocyanate
TDL	thoracic-duct lymphocytes
TDM	therapeutic drug monitoring
TDN	totally digestible nutrients

tds	to be taken three times a day *(ter die sumendum)*
TdT	terminal deoxynucleotidyl transferase
TDT	tone decay test
t$_e$	effective half-life
Te	tellurium • tetanus
TE	tracheoesophageal • trial and error
T&E	trial and error
TEA	tetraethylammonium
TEAB	tetraethylammonium bromide
TEAC	tetraethylammonium chloride
TEAE	triethylaminoethyl
TeBG	testosterone-binding globulin
TEC	total eosinophil count
tech	technical • technique
TED	threshold erythema dose
TEDS	thromboembolus deterrent stocking
TEE	thermal effect of exercise • transesophageal echocardiogram
TEF	thermal effect of food
t$_{eff}$	effective half-life
TEFRA	Tax Equity and Fiscal Responsibility Act
TEG	thromboelastogram, thromboelastography
TEL	tetraethyl lead
TEM	transmission electron microscope • triethylenemelamine
temp	temperature • temporary
temp dext	to the right temple *(tempori dextro)*
temp sinist	to the left temple *(tempori sinistro)*
TEN	total enteral nutrition • toxic epidermal necrolysis

TENS	transcutaneous electrical nerve stimulator
TEPA	triethylenephosphoramide
TEPP	tetraethyl pyrophosphate
ter	rub *(tere)*
Terb	terbutaline
term	terminal
tert	tertiary
TES	treatment of emergent symptom
TET	treadmill exercise test
TETD	disulfiram (tetraethylthiuram disulfide)
TETRAC	tetraiodothyroacetic acid
tet tox	tetanus toxoid
tf	to follow • tuning fork
Tf	transferrin
TF	transfer factor
TFA	total fatty acids
TFB	trifascicular block
TFS	testicular feminization syndrome
TFT	thyroid function test
tg	type genus
Tg	thyroglobulin
TG	thioguanine • thyroglobulin • toxic goiter • triglyceride • type genus
TGA	transient global amnesia
TGF-α	type alpha-transforming growth factor
TGF-β	transforming growth factor - beta
TGE	transmissible gastroenteritis • tryptone glucose extract
TGFA	triglyceride fatty acid

TGT	thromboplastin generation test • thromboplastin generation time
TGV	thoracic gas volume
th	thoracic
Th	thorium
TH	tube holder
THA	tetrahydroaminoacridine • total hip arthroplasty • total hydroxyapatite
THAM	tris(hydroxymethyl)aminomethane
THC	tetrahydrocannabinol • transhepatic cholangiogram, cholangiography
ther	therapeutic • therapy
Ther Ex	therapeutic exercise
therm	thermometer
THF	tetrahydrofluorenone • tetrahydrofolate • tetrahydrofuran
THFA	tetrahydrofolic acid
Thg	thyroglobulin
THI	trihydroxyindole
thor	thorax, thoracic
Thr	threonine
THR	total hip replacement
throm	thrombosis
THS	terahydro-compound S • tetrahydrodeoxycortisol
THU	tetrahydrouridine
Ti	titanium
TI	transverse diameter between ischia • tricuspid incompetence • tricuspid insufficiency
TIA	transient ischemic attack
TIBC	total iron-binding capacity

tib-fib	tibia and fibula
TIC	trypsin inhibitory capacity
tid	three times a day *(ter in die)*
TID	titrated initial dose
TIG	tetanus immune globulin
tin	three times a night *(ter in nocte)*
TIN	tubulointerstitial nephropathy
tinct	tincture
TIP	Terbutaline infusion pump
TIR	terminal innervation ratio
TIRI	total immunoreactive insulin
TISS	Therapeutic Intervention Scoring System
Title XVII	Medicare
Title XIX	Medicaid
tiwk	three times a week
TJ	triceps jerk
TK	through the knee • tourniquet • transketolase
TKD	tokodynamometer
TKG	tokodynagraph
TKO	to keep open
Tl	thallium
TL	team leader • tubal ligation
T/L	terminal latency (EMG)
TLC	tender loving care • thin-layer chro- matography • total lung capacity • total lymphocyte count
TLD	thermoluminescent dosimeter • transluminescent dosimeter
TLE	thin-layer electrophoresis
TLI	total lymphoid irradiation

TLR	tonic labyrinthine reflex
TLSO	thoracolumbosacral orthosis
TLV	threshold limit value • total lung volume
Tm	maximum (maximal) tubular excretory capacity • thulium
TM	temporomandibular • Thayer- Martin (medium) • trademark • Transcendental Meditation • transport mechanism • trimester • tympanic membrane
TMB	too many birthdays
TmG	maximum (maximal) tubular glucose reabsorption rate
TMI	threatened myocardial infarction
TMJ	temporomandibular joint (syndrome)
TML	tetramethyl lead
TMP	thymidine monophosphate • trimethoprim • trimethylpsoralen
TMP-SMX	trimethoprim-sulfamethoxazole
TMP-SMZ	trimethoprim-sulfamethoxazole
TMP-SMZ-DS	trimethoprim-sulfamethoxazole - double strength
TMT	tympanic membrane thermometer
TMV	tobacco mosaic virus
Tn	normal intraocular tension
TN	true-negative
TNBP	tri(n-butyl) phosphate
TNCC	trauma nursing core course
TNF	tumor necrosis factor
TNG	nitroglycerin (trinitroglycerol)
TNI	total nodal irradiation
TNM	tumor, nodes, metastases
TNPM	transient neonatal pustular melanosis

TNS	transcutaneous electrical nerve stimulator
TNT	trinitrotoluene
TNTC	too numerous to count
TO	original tuberculin • target organ • telephone order • temperature, oral • Theiler's Original (virus) • tincture of opium
TOA	time of arrival • tubo-ovarian abscess
TOCP	triorthocresyl phosphate
tol	tolerance
tomo	tomogram, tomography
tonoc	tonight
top	topical , topically
TOP	termination of pregnancy
TOPS	Total Ozone Portable Spectrometer
TOPV	trivalent oral poliovirus vaccine
TORCH	*Toxoplasma*, rubella, cytomegalovirus, herpes simplex (screen)
TORP	total ossicular replacement prosthesis
TOTAL-C	total cholesterol
tourn	tourniquet
tox	toxic, toxicity, toxicology
t$_p$	physical half-life
TP	toilet paper • total protein • *Treponema pallidum* • true-positive
tPA	tissue plasminogen activator
TPA	third party administrator • tissue plasminogen activator
TPC	thromboplastic plasma component
TPCF	*Treponema pallidum* complement fixation (test)
TPE	therapeutic plasma exchange (plasmapheresis)

TPH	thromboembolic pulmonary hypertension
TPHA	*Treponema pallidum* hemagglutination (test)
TPi	*Treponema pallidum* immobilization (test)
TPIA	*Treponema pallidum* immune adherence
TPM	temporary pacemaker
TPN	total parenteral nutrition • triphosphopyridine nucleotide
TPNH	triphosphopyridine nucleotide reduced form
TPO	tryptophan peroxidase
TPP	thiamine pyrophosphate
TPR	temperature, pulse and respiration • testosterone production rate • total peripheral resistance • total pulmonary resistance
TPVR	total peripheral vascular resistance
TQM	total quality management
t_r	radiologic half-life
tr	tincture • trace • traction • treatment • tremor
TR	new tuberculin (tuberculin residue) • severe trauma • temperature, rectal • therapeutic radiology • tricuspid regurgitation • tubular resorption • turbidity-reducing
trach	trachea • tracheostomy
trans	transverse
transm	transmission
transpl	transplant
trans sect	transverse section
TRAP	tartrate-resistant leukocyte acid phosphatase
TRBF	total renal blood flow
TRC	tanned red cell
treat	treatment
Trend	Trendelenburg (position, cannula, etc.)

Trep	*Treponema*
TRF	T-cell replacing factor • thyrotropin-releasing factor
TRH	thyrotropin-releasing hormone
TRI	total response index • trifocal
TRIC	trachoma-inclusion conjunctivitis
Trich	*Trichomonas*
trid	three days *(tridium)*
Trig	triglycerides
TRIS	tris (hydroxymethyl) aminomethane
TRIT	triturate
tRNA	transfer ribonucleic acid
TRO	temporary restraining order
Trp	tryptophan
TRP	tubular resorption of phosphate
TRS	tuboreticular structures
TRT	treatment
TRU	turbidity-reducing unit
T$_3$RU	triiodothyronine resin uptake
Tryp	tryptophan
TS	terminal sensation • test solution • thoracic surgery • tracheal sound • tricuspid stenosis • triple-strength • tubular sound
T/S	thyroid-serum iodide ratio
TSA	trypticase soy agar • tumor-specific antigen
TSBB	transtracheal selective bronchial brushing
TSD	target-to-skin distance • Tay-Sachs disease
TSF	thrombopoietic-stimulating factor • triceps skin fold
TSG	tumor suppression gene
TSH	thyroid-stimulating hormone

TSH-RF	thyroid-stimulating hormone-releasing factor
TSI	thyroid-stimulating immunoglobulin • triple sugar iron (agar)
TSIA	triple sugar iron agar
tsp	teaspoonful
TSP	total serum protein
T-spica	thumb spica (bandage, cast)
T-spine	thoracic spine
TSR	transfer
TSS	toxic shock syndrome
TST	tumor skin test
TSTA	tumor-specific transplantation antigen
TT	tetanus toxoid • therapeutic touch • thrombin time • thymol turbidity (test) • transit time (blood through heart)
TT$_4$	total (serum) thyroxine
TTA	transtracheal aspirates
TTC	triphenyltetrazolium chloride
TTH	thyrotropic hormone
TTI	tension-time index • tissue thromboplastin inhibition (test)
TTM	transtelephonic ECG monitoring
TTN	transient tachypnea of the newborn
TTNB	transient tachypnea of the newborn
TTP	therapeutic touch practitioner • thrombotic thrombocytopenic purpura • thymidine triphosphate
TTS	temporary threshold shift
TU	toxin unit • transmission unit • tuberculin unit
T$_3$U	triiodothyronine resin uptake (test)
tuberc	tuberculosis, tuberculous

TUR	transurethral resection
T3UR	triiodothyronine uptake ratio
turb	turbidity
TURB	transurethral resection of the bladder
TURBTs	transurethral resection of bladder tumors
TURP	transurethral resection of the prostate
tus	cough *(tussis)*
tv	transvenous
TV	television • tetrazolium violet • tidal volume • total volume • trial visit • *Trichomonas vaginalis*
TVC	timed vital capacity • true vocal cord
TVH	total vaginal hysterectomy
TVR	tonic vibration reflex
TW	thin-walled
TWB	touch weight-bearing
TWE	tap-water enema
Tx	traction • transplant • treatment
TXA$_2$	thromboxane A$_2$
TXB$_2$	thromboxane B$_2$
Ty	type
Tyr	tyrosine

U

U	unit • upper • uracil • uranium • urine • urology, urologist
U100	100 units per millimeter
ua	up to, as far as *(usque ad)*
UA	uric acid • urinalysis • urocanic acid
U/A	urinalysis • uterine activity
UAC	umbilical artery catheter
UAGA	Uniform Anatomical Gift Act
UAI	uterine activity integral
UAL	up (out of bed) as desired *(ad lbiitum)*
UAO	upper airway obstruction
UAP	unlicensed assistive personnel
UAT	up (out of bed) as tolerated
UB	Unna's boot
UB-82	Uniform Billing Form of 1982
UBA	undenatured bacterial antigen
UBG	urobilinogen
UBI	ultraviolet blood irradiation
UC	ulcerative colitis • Uldall catheter • unchanged • unit coordinator • urea clearance • urinary catheter • usual care • uterine contractions
UCA	unit communications assistant
UCC	urgent care center
UCD	usual childhood diseases
UCG	urinary chorionic gonadotropin

UCHD	usual childhood diseases
UCL	uncomfortable loudness level • urea clearance
UCNT	undifferentiated carcinoma of the nasopharyngeal type
UCPA	United Cerebral Palsy Associations
UCR	unconditioned reflex • unconditioned response • usual, customary and reasonable
UCR/ PACE	usual, customary and reasonable/performance and cost efficiency
UCS	unconditioned stimulus
UCV	uncontrolled variable
ud	as directed *(ut dictum)*
UD	unipolar depression • urethral discharge • uridine diphosphate
UDC	usual diseases of childhood
UDCA	ursodeoxycholic acid
UDO	undetermined origin
UDP	uridine diphosphate
UDPG	uridine diphosphoglucose
UDPGA	uridine disphosphoglucuronic acid
UDPGT	urine diphosphoglucuronyl- transferase
UE	upper extremity
UES	upper esophageal sphincter
UF	ultrafiltration
UFA	unesterified fatty acids
UG	urogenital
UGA	under general anesthesia
UGDP	University Group Diabetes Program
UGH	uveitis, glaucoma, hyphema
UGI	upper gastrointestinal

UGI-SB	upper gastrointestinal, small bowel
UGI-SBFT	upper gastrointestinal with small bowel follow-through (x-ray)
UHDDS	Uniform Hospital Discharge Data Set
UHF	ultrahigh frequency
UHV	ultrahigh voltage
UI	uroporphyrin isomerase
UIBC	unsaturated iron-binding capacity
UK	urokinase
U/L	upper and lower
ULQ	upper left quadrant
ult	ultimate, ultimately
ult praes	at last prescribed *(ultimum praescriptus)*
UM	upper motor (neuron) • uracil mustard • uterine monitor • Utilization Management
umb	umbilical, umbilicus
UMP	uridine monophosphate
UN	urea nitrogen
U$_{NA}$	urine sodium
uncomp	uncompensated
uncond	unconditioned
uncond ref	unconditioned reflex
uncor	uncorrected
unCS	unconditioned stimulus
ung	ointment *(unguentum)*
unilat	unilateral, unilaterally
univ	university
unk	unknown
UNOS	United Network for Organ Sharing

UnS	unconditioned stimulus
UNSCEAR	United Nations Scientific Committee on the Effects of Atomic Radiation
UOP	urinary output
UOQ	upper outer quadrant
UOS	unit of service
UP	ureteropelvic • uteroplacental
U/P	ratio of urine concentration to plasma concentration
up ad lib	up (out of bed) as desired (*ad libitum*)
UPI	uteroplacental insufficiency
UPJ	ureteropelvic junction
UPP	urethral pressure profilometry
UPRR	unit peer recognition and reward
UQ	upper quadrant
ur	urine
UR	unconditioned reflex • unconditioned response • unrelated • upper respiratory • utilization review
URC	utilization review committee • utilization review coordinator
Urd	uridine
URI	upper respiratory infection
Urol	urology, urologist
URQ	upper right quadrant
URTI	upper respiratory tract infection
US	ultrasonic, ultrasonography, ultrasound • unconditioned stimulus • unit secretary
U/S	ultrasound
USAEC	United States Atomic Energy Commission
USAN	United States Adopted Name
USD	United States Dispensatory

USN	ultrasonic nebulization, nebulizer • United States Navy
USNH	United States Naval Hospital
USP	United States Pharmacopeia
USPC	United States Pharmacopeial Convention
USPHS	United States Public Health Service
USR	unheated serum reagin
USRDA	United States Recommended Dietary Allowance
UTBG	unbound thyroxine-binding globulin
ut dict	as directed *(ut dictum)*
utend	to be used *(utendus)*
UTI	urinary tract infection
UTP	uridine triphosphate
UTZ	ultrasound
UU	urine urobilinogen
UUN	urine urea nitrogen
UV	ultraviolet
UVA	long-wavelength ultraviolet light (320-400 nm)
UVB	medium-wavelength ultraviolet light (290-320 nm)
UVC	short-wavelength ultraviolet light (less than 290 nm)
UVJ	ureterovesical junction
UVL	ultraviolet light
UVR	ultraviolet radiation
UWS	underwater seal (drainage)
UZ	ultrasound

V

v	see *(vide)* • vein • velocity • venous blood • volt
V	unipolar ECG chest lead (V1, V2,...V6) • vanadium • vein • velocity • venous blood • ventilation • verbal • vertex • *Vibrio* • viral, virus • virulence • vision • visual acuity • visual capacity • voice • volt • volume
V°	gas volume per unit of time
va	volt-ampere
Va	arterial gas volume
VA	alveolar gas volume • vacuum aspiration • ventriculoatrial • Veterans Administration • visual acuity • volt-ampere
vac	vacuum
VAC	vincristine, actinomycin D, cyclophosphamide
vacc	vaccination
VACTERL	vertebral, anal, cardiac, tracheoesophageal, renal, limb (syndrome)
VAD	ventricular assistive device • vincristine, adriamycin, dexamethasone
VAE	venous air embolism
vag	vagina, vaginal
Vag Hyst	vaginal hysterectomy
VAH	Veterans Administration Hospital
VAHS	virus-associated hemophagocytic syndrome
val	valine • valve
VAMC	Veterans Administration Medical Center
VAMP	vincristine, amethopterin, 6-mercaptopurine, prednisone

VAP	ventilator-associated pneumonia
V°a/Q°c	ratio of ventilation (alveolar) to perfusion (pulmonary capillary)
var	variation, variety
vasc	vascular
VASC	Verbal Auditory Screen for Children
vasodil	vasodilation
VAT	ventricular pacing, atrial sensing, triggered mode (pacemaker)
VATER	vertebral, anal, tracheoesophageal fistula, and radial or renal (deficiencies)
VATH	vinblastine, adriamycin, thiotepa, halotestin
VATS	video-assisted thoracoscopic surgery
VB	vinblastine
VBAC	vaginal birth after cesarean
VBG	venoaortocoronary artery bypass graft • vertical banded gastroplasty
VBI	vertebrobasilar insufficiency
VBM	vinblastine, bleomycin, methotrexate
V$_c$	pulmonary capillary gas volume
VC	acuity of color vision • capillary volume • vena cava • venous capacitance • ventilatory capacity • vincristine • vital capacity • vocal cord
VCA	viral capsid antigen
V$_{CF}$	mean fiber-shortening rate
VCG	vectorcardiogram
VCM	vinyl chloride monomer
VCO$_2$	carbon dioxide output
V°CO$_2$	carbon dioxide output rate
VCR	vincristine
VCU	voiding cystourethrogram

vd	double vibrations
V$_D$	dead-space gas volume
VD	venereal disease
VDA	venous digital angiogram • visual discriminatory acuity
VDC	vasodilator center
VDEL	Venereal Disease Experimental Laboratory
VDG	venereal disease - gonorrhea
VDH	valvular disease of the heart
VDM	vasodepressor material
VDRL	Venereal Disease Research Laboratory (test)
VDS	vasodilator substance • venereal disease - syphilis
VDT	video display terminal
VDU	visual display unit
V$_D$/V$_T$	ratio of dead-space gas volume to tidal gas volume
V$_E$	volume of expired gas
VE	vesicular exanthem • visual examination
VEA	ventricular ectopic arrhythmia
vect	vector
VEE	Venezuelan equine encephalitis • Venezuelan equine encephalomyelitis
vel	velocity
VEM	vasoexcitor material
vent	ventilation, ventilator • ventral • ventricle, ventricular
vent fib	ventricular fibrillation
VEP	visual evoked potential
VER	visual evoked response
vert	vertebra • vertical
ves	bladder *(vesica)* • vesicular

vesic	bladder *(vesica)*
VETS	Veterans Adjustment Scale
VF	ventricular fibrillation • ventricular flutter • video frequency • visual field • vocal fremitus
VFC	ventricular function curve
VFD	visual feed-back display
VFib	ventricular fibrillation
v flutter	ventricular flutter
VF/VT	ventricular fibrillation and ventricular tachycardia
VG	vein graft • ventricular gallop • very good
VH	vaginal hysterectomy • veterans hospital • viral hepatitis
VHDL	very high density lipoprotein
VHF	very high frequency
VHL	Von Hippel-Lindau disease
V$_I$	volume of inspired gas
VI	volume index
VIA	virus-inactivating agent
vib	vibration
VIC	vasoinhibitory center
vid	see *(vide)*
VIG	vaccinia immune globulin
vin	wine *(vinum)*
VIP	vasoactive intestinal polypeptide • very important person
VIQ	Verbal Intelligence Quotient
vis	vision • visiting, visitor
VIS	vaginal irrigation smear
visc	visceral • viscous, viscosity
vit	vital • vitamin

vitel	yolk *(vitellus)*
viz	that is, namely *(videlicet)*
VLBW	very low birth weight
VLCD	very low calorie diet
VLDL	very low density lipoprotein
VLDL-TG	very low density lipoprotein - triglyceride
VLF	very low frequency
VLM	visceral larva migrans
VLP	ventriculolumbar perfusion
VM	Venturi mask • viomycin • voltmeter
VMA	vanillylmandelic acid
V$_{max}$	maximum velocity, rate
VNA	Visiting Nurse Association
VNS	Visiting Nurse Service
VO	verbal order
VO$_2$	oxygen consumption
V°O$_2$	oxygen consumption rate
VOD	vision, right eye *(oculus dexter)*
vol	volume
VOO	ventricular pacing, no sensing, no other function (pacemaker)
VOS	vision, left eye *(oculus sinister)*
VOT	Visual Organization Test
VOU	vision, each eye *(oculus sinister)*
vp	vapor pressure
VP	variegate porphyria • vasopressin • venipuncture • venous pressure • ventriculo-peritoneal shunt • Voges-Proskauer reaction
V&P	vagotomy and pyloroplasty
VPA	valproic acid

VPB	ventricular premature beat
VPC	ventricular premature contraction
VPD	ventricular premature depolarization
VPI	velopharyngeal insufficiency
VPN	Vice-President, Nursing
V°/Q°	ventilation-perfusion ratio
VR	right vision • variable ratio • venous return • ventilation rate • ventral root (of spinal nerves) • ventricular response • vocal resonance • vocational rehabilitation
VRA	Vocational Rehabilitation Administration
VR&E	vocational rehabilitation and education
VRI	viral respiratory infection
VRP	very reliable product
VRV	ventricular residual volume
vs	single vibrations • versus • vibration-second
VS	ventricular septum • vesicular sound • vesicular stomatitis • vital signs • volumetric solution
VSD	ventricular septal defect
VSR	venous stasis retinopathy
V_t	pulmonary parenchymal tissue volume
V_T	tidal gas volume
VT	ventricular tachycardia
V&T	volume and tension
vtach	ventricular tachycardia
VTE	venous thromboembolism • vicarious trial and error
V_{TG}	thoracic gas volume
VTI	volume thickness index
VTR	videotape recording
VTSRS	Verdun Target Symptom Rating Scale

VTT	video tape training
vtx	vertex
VUR	vesicoureteral reflux • vesicoureteral regurgitation
vv	veins
VV	varicose veins • vulva and vagina
v/v	vice versa • volume (of solute) per volume (of solvent)
VVI	ventricular pacing, ventricular sensing, inhibited mode (pacemaker)
VVT	ventricular pacing, ventricular sensing, triggered mode (pacemaker)
VW	vessel wall
V/W	volume of a substance per unit of weight of another component
vWF	von Willebrand factor
VWF	von Willebrand factor
VWFT	variable-width forms tractor
Vx	vertex
VZ	varicella-zoster
VZID	varicella-zoster immune globulin disease
VZIG	varicella-zoster immune globulin
VZV	varicella-zoster virus

W

w	watt • week • wife • with
W	tungsten *(wolfram)* • water • watt • weber (unit of magnetic flux) • wehnelt unit • weight • white cell • widow, widowed, widower • width • word fluency
WA	when awake
WAIS	Wechsler Adult Intelligence Scale
WAIS-R	Wechsler Adult Intelligence Scale - Revised
WAP	wandering atrial pacemaker
Wass	Wassermann test
Wb	weber (unit of magnetic flux)
WB	washable base • water bottle • Wechsler-Bellevue (scale) • weight-bearing • wet-bulb • whole blood
WBAT	weight-bearing as tolerated
WBC	white blood cell • white blood (cell) count
WBCT	whole-blood clotting time
WBH	whole-body hematocrit
WBPTT	whole-blood partial thromboplastin time
WBR	whole body radiation
WBS	whole body scan
WBT	wet-bulb temperature
w/c	wheelchair
WC	ward clerk • water closet (bathroom) • wheelchair • whooping cough
WCGS	Western Collaborative Group Study
WCR	Walthard's cell rests

wd	ward • wound
WD	well-developed • well-differentiated • wet dressing • Wilson's disease • wrist disarticulation
w/d	warm and dry • well-developed
WDHA	watery diarrhea, hypokalemia, achlorhydria
WD/WN	well-developed, well-nourished
W/E	week-end
WEE	Western equine encephalitis • Western equine encephalomyelitis
wf	white female
WFL	within functional limits
wh	whisper, whispered • white
WH	well-healed • well-hydrated
WHO	World Health Organization
w-hr	watt-hour
WHVP	wedged hepatic venous pressure
WIA	wounded in action
WIC	Welfare and Institution Code • women, infants and children
wid	widow, widowed, widower
WISC	Wechsler Intelligence Scale for Children
WISC-R	Wechsler Intelligence Scale for Children - Revised
wk	weak • week
WK	Wernicke-Korsakoff (syndrome)
/wk	per week
WL	waiting list • wavelength • work load
WLM	working-level month
wm	white male
WM	wall motion • wet mount • whole milk • whole mount

WMA	World Medical Association
WMS	wall-motion study • Wechsler Memory Scale
Wms. Flex. Ex.	Williams flexion exercises
w/n	well-nourished
WN	well-nourished
wnd	wound
WNL	within normal limits
wo	weeks old
w/o	without
W/O	water in oil
WOR	Weber-Osler-Rondu (syndrome)
WOU	women's outpatient unit
w/p	whirlpool
WP	wet pack • working point
WPPSI	Wechsler Preschool and Primary Scale of Intelligence
WPW	Wolf-Parkinson-White (syndrome)
WR	Wassermann reaction • work rate
WRAT	Wide-Range Achievement Test
ws	watt second
WS	ward secretary • water-soluble
WSD	water seal drainage
wt	weight
w/u	work-up
w/v	weight (of solute) per volume (of solvent)
WV	whispered voice
w/w	weight (of solute) per weight (of solvent)

X

x	axis • multiplied by • times
X	cross • cross section • Kienböck's unit (of X-ray exposure) • multiplied by • times • transverse section • unknown
x̄	mean
X̄	except
Xa	chiasma
Xao	xanthosine
XC	excretory cystogram
XD	X-linked dominant
XDP	xeroderma pigmentosum
Xe	xenon
Xfmr	transformer
XGP	xanthogranulomatous pyelonephritis
XLP	X-linked lymphoproliferative (disorder)
X-match	crossmatch
XMP	xanthosine monophosphate
XO	xanthine oxidase
XP	exophoria • xeroderma pigmentosum
XR	X-linked recessive • x-ray
XRT	X-ray therapy
XT	exotropia, exotropic
XU	excretory urogram
XUV	extreme ultraviolet
XX	normal female sex chromosome type

XY	normal male sex chromosome type
Xyl	xylose
Xylo	Xylocaine

Y

y	yield
Y	young • yttrium
YACP	young adult chronic patient
YAG	yttrium-aluminum-garnet (laser)
Yb	ytterbium
yd	yard
YE	yellow enzyme
yel	yellow
YF	yellow fever
y/o	years old
YOB	year of birth
YP	yeast phase • yield pressure
yr	year
ys	yellow spot
YS	yolk sac
YTD	year-to-date

Z

Z	no effect • symbol for atomic number • zero • zone
Z, Z′, Z″	increasing degrees of contraction
ZDV	zidovudine
ZE	Zollinger-Ellison (syndrome)
ZES	Zollinger-Ellison syndrome
ZIG	zoster immune globulin
ZIP	zoster immune plasma
Zn	zinc
Zn fl	zinc flocculation (test)
ZPG	zero population growth
Zr	zirconium
ZSR	zeta sedimentation rate • zinc sedimentation rate
Zz	ginger *(zingiber)*

EPONYMS

Abadie sign

spasm of the levator palpebrae superioris in thyrotoxicosis.

Aberhalden-Kauffman-Lignac syndrome

renal rickets with cystinosis.

Achard-Thiers syndrome

women with diabetes and aspects of both adrenogenital syndrome and Cushing syndrome including masculinization and menstrual disorders.

Achilles tendon

the tendon attaching the gastrocnemius to the calcaneus.

Ackerman tumor

verrucous carcinoma of the larynx.

Acosta disease

hypoxic disease caused by high elevation.

Addison disease

syndrome caused by insufficient hormone production by the adrenal glands.

Adson test

a test for thoracic outlet syndrome.

Albright syndrome

an inherited hypoparathyroidism associated with skeletal defects; polyostotic fibrous dysplasia.

Alcock canal

a tunnel enclosing pudendal vessels and nerves.

Alpers disease

progressive cerebral poliodystrophy.

Alzheimer disease

irreversible degenerative senile dementia.

Ames test

a test for carcinogens using strains of *Salmonella typhinium* that will mutate if carcinogens are present.

Anders disease

adiposa tuberosa simplex.

Andersen disease

type IV glycogenosis.

Andersen syndrome

cystic fibrosis of the pancreas, bronchiectasis and vitamin A deficiency.

Apert syndrome

acrocephalosyndactyly, type I.

Apert-Crouzon disease

acrocephalosyndactyly, type I.

Apgar score

a numerical score evaluating the condition of an infant at birth.

Aran-Duchenne disease

spinal muscular atrophy.

Argyll Robertson pupil

a miotic pupil which reacts to accommodation but does not react to light.

Arnold ganglion

otic ganglion, situated below the foramen ovale medial to the mandibular nerve.

Arnold-Chiari deformity (malformation/syndrome)

congenital anomaly of the cerebellum and medulla oblongata.

Arnold Pick disease (atrophy)

circumscribed cerebral atrophy.

Ascheim-Zondek test

a pregnancy test performed by injecting the woman's urine into immature female mice.

Aschoff bodies (nodules)

granuloma specific for rheumatic fever.

Ashman phenomenon

an aberrant arrhythmia of atrial fibrillation.

Auer bodies

faulty granule formations in myeloblastic and monoblastic leukemia.

Auerbach plexus

esophageal autonomic nerve plexus.

Austin Flint murmur

diastolic mitral valve murmur.

Ayerza disease (syndrome)

a type of polycythemia vera.

Babès-Ernst granules (bodies)

metachromatic granules present in bacterial cells, yeasts, fungi and protozoa.

Babington disease

hereditary telangiectasia.

Babinski reflex (sign)

dorsiflexion of the great toe upon plantar stimulation, considered indicative of pyramidal tract disturbance.

Baghdad boil

a lesion occurring in cutaneous leishmaniasis.

Baker cyst

enlarged popliteal bursa associated with degenerative disease of the knee.

Balser fatty necrosis

gangrenous pancreatitis with omental bursitis and disseminated patches of necrosis of the fatty tissues.

Bamberger-Marie disease

hypertrophic pulmonary osteoarthropathy.

Banti disease (syndrome)

portal hypertension with congestive splenomegaly.

Barlow disease

infantile scurvy.

Barlow syndrome

mitral valve prolapse syndrome.

Barr body

sex chromatin.

Barrett esophagus (syndrome)

chronic peptic ulcer of the lower esophagus.

Bartholin cyst

a retention cyst of the major vestibular or Bartholin gland.

Bartholin gland

greater vestibular gland; vulvovaginal gland.

Barton fracture

a fracture of the distal radius into the wrist joint.

Bartter syndrome

juxtaglomerular cell hyperplasia with hypokalemic alkalosis and hyperaldosteronism.

Basedow disease

Graves' disease; a form of hyperthyroidism characterized by thyrotoxicosis with diffuse hyperplasia, exophthalmos or pretibial myxedema.

Bassen-Kornzweig syndrome

abetalipoproteinemia.

Battle sign

discoloration near the tip of the mastoid process which is seen in basilar skull fractures.

Beau lines

transverse grooves on fingernails after serious illness or trauma.

Behçet syndrome

chronic inflammatory disorder involving ulcerations of mucous membranes in the mouth, genitals and eyes, and frequently arthritis.

Bell's palsy

paralysis of the facial nerve.

Bence Jones protein

an abnormal protein found in the urine of patients with multiple myeloma.

Benedict solution

an aqueous solution of sodium citrate, sodium carbonate and copper sulfate that is used to test for the presence of glucose in the urine.

Berger disease

glomerulonephritis.

Bernheim syndrome

right ventricular failure with left ventricular hypertrophy.

Billroth gastrectomy (operation)

resection of the stomach with anastomosis to the duodenum (Billroth I) or to the jejunum (Billroth II).

Blackfan-Diamond anemia

congenital hypoplastic anemia.

Blalock-Taussig operation

surgery to repair the congenital cardiac defect known as the tetralogy of Fallot.

Braxton-Hicks contractions

light, painless uterine contractions during pregnancy.

Bright disease

chronic nonsuppurative nephritis.

Broca aphasia

also termed ataxic, expressive or motor aphasia; patients with Broca's aphasia have difficulty with verbal expression and articulation, but may write or sign well.

Brompton solution (cocktail)

an analgesic cocktail usually of morphine and cocaine often given to the terminally ill.

Brunner glands

duodenal glands.

Budd-Chiari syndrome

hepatosplenomegaly, jaundice, ascites and portal hypertension caused by hepatic vein occlusion.

Burkitt's lymphoma

a malignant lymphoma usually found in Africa, but also seen elsewhere including the United States, that may involve the facial bones, ovaries, or abdominal lymph nodes.

Chadwick sign

a blue discoloration of vaginal mucosa that indicates pregnancy.

Charcot-Marie-Tooth disease

peroneal muscular atrophy.

Cheyne-Stokes respirations

recurrent episodes of rapid breathing alternating with apnea, often seen in coma resulting from affection of the nervous centers.

Christmas disease

hemophilia B; also called Factor IX deficiency (hemophilia); caused by hereditary deficiency of Factor IX.

Colles fracture

fractured distal radius with posterior displacement.

Coombs test

antiglobulin test.

Cowper cyst

retention cyst of the bulbourethral glands.

Crohn's disease

regional ileitis or enteritis.

Cushing syndrome

hyperadrenocorticism; also called Cushing's basophilism or pituitary basophilism.

Dakin solution (fluid)

antiseptic of diluted sodium hypochlorite used to irrigate wounds.

Down syndrome

a syndrome of mental retardation caused by a chromosomal abnormality where chromosome 21 appears three times instead of twice in some or all cells. Also called trisomy 21; formerly called mongolism.

Duchenne paralysis

(1) progressive bulbar paralysis; (2) pseudohypertrophic muscular dystrophy.

Dupuytren contracture

flexure of the 4th and 5th fingers due to contracture of palmar fascia.

Eddowes disease (syndrome)

osteogenesis imperfecta.

Ehlers-Danlos syndrome

cutis hyperelastica; a group of inherited connective tissue disorders producing overelasticity and friability of the skin, excessive extensibility of the joints, and fragility of the cutaneous blood vessels, due to deficient quality or quantity of collagen.

Epstein-Barr virus

a virus found in infectious mononucleosis and Burkitt's lymphoma; human herpesvirus 4.

Erb-Goldflam disease

myasthenia gravis.

Ewing sarcoma

malignant bone tumor usually found in children.

Fallot tetralogy

ventricular-septal defect, pulmonary stenosis, right ventricular hypertrophy and dextraposition of the aorta occurring as a congenital anomaly.

Friedländer bacillus

Klebsiella pneumoniae.

Friedreich ataxia

hereditary spinal ataxia; an autosomal recessive disease usually beginning in childhood with sclerosis of the posterior and lateral columns of the spinal cord and ataxia of the lower extremities, followed by paralysis and contractures.

Gifford sign

inability to evert the upper eyelid in Graves' disease (hyperthyroidism).

Goodpasture syndrome

acute glomerulonephritis with intrapulmonary hemorrhage, hemoptysis and anemia, usually progressing to renal failure.

Graves' disease

a form of hyperthyroidism characterized by diffuse goiter, often seen with exophthalmos.

Guillain-Barré syndrome

acute idiopathic polyneuritis; rapidly progressing ascending motor neuron paralysis usually beginning with the feet and spreading to the legs, arms, trunk and face.

Gull disease

atrophy of the thyroid with myxedema (hypothyroidism).

Hand-Schüller-Christian disease

chronic idiopathic histiocytosis.

Hansen disease

leprosy.

Hartmann pouch

abnormal pouch formed at the neck of the gallbladder.

Hartmann solution

intravenous lactated Ringer's solution.

Hashimoto disease

autoimmune thyroiditis.

Heberden nodes

bony prominence and flexion deformities of the finger joints associated with osteoarthritis.

Heimlich maneuver

a method of dislodging a foreign body from the airway by applying quick thrust pressure to the subdiaphragmatic area.

Hirschberg sign

adduction reflex of the foot.

Hirschsprung disease

congenital megacolon.

Hodgkin disease

a common malignant lymphoma marked by chronic enlargement of the lymph nodes together with enlargement of the spleen and often liver.

Hodgson disease

uniform aneurysmal dilatation of the aorta associated with insufficiency of the aortic valve, often accompanied by dilatation or hypertrophy of the heart.

Homans' sign

pain upon passive dorsiflexion of the foot as a positive sign for deep venous thrombus.

Horton syndrome (cephalalgia)

histaminic or cluster headache.

Huntington chorea

hereditary chorea; autosomal dominant disease characterized by irregular, spasmodic movements in the face and extremities, accompanied by progressive mental deterioration ending in dementia.

Hurler disease (syndrome)

mucopolysaccharidosis IH.

Ishihara test

a test for color blindness that utilizes plates upon which figures are formed from round dots of various colors.

Jakob-Creutzfeldt disease

spastic pseudoparalysis; a rare, usually fatal, transmissible spongiform encephalopathy characterized by progressive dementia, myoclonus and ataxia.

Kawasaki syndrome (disease)

febrile mucocutaneous lymph node disease.

Kaposi sarcoma

multiple idiopathic hemorrhagic sarcoma; multifocal malignant neoplasm characterized by reddish-purple cutaneous lesions, usually seen in men over 60 years of age and as an opportunistic infection in AIDS patients.

Kernig sign

flexion of hip and extension of leg while recumbent causes pain; a positive sign for meningitis.

Kirschner wire (apparatus)

a steel wire used for skeletal fixation of, and obtaining skeletal traction in, fractures.

Klinefelter syndrome

XXY syndrome; feminization of males due to extra X chromosomes combined with one Y chromosome, resulting in small testes and infertility.

Koenig syndrome (König)

diarrhea alternating with constipation, seen with abdominal pain, meteorism and gurgling sounds on the right iliac fossa, symptomatic of cecal tuberculosis.

Krebs cycle

citric acid or tricarboxylic acid cycle; a basic metabolic mechanism involving the oxidation of acetic acid for energy stored in phosphate bonds.

Kussmaul disease

polyarteritis nodosa; necrosis of the small and medium-sized arteries.

Kussmal respirations

rapid, deep respiration due to diabetic ketoacidosis.

Laënnec cirrhosis

alcoholic micronodular cirrhosis in which normal liver nodules are replaced by small regeneration nodules, sometimes containing fat.

Langerhans adenoma

an islet cell adenoma of the pancreas; insulinoma.

Langerhans, Isles of

pancreatic insulin- and glucagon-producing cell clusters or islets.

Legg-Calvé-Perths disease

osteochondritis deformans juvenilis; necrosis of the upper end of the femur.

Lhermitte sign

flexing the neck forward causes electric-shock-like pain in the extremities as a sign of multiple sclerosis or compression and other disorders of the cervical cord.

Lyme disease

recurrent multisystemic disorder caused by a tick-borne spirochete characterized by erythema chronicum migrans lesions, fever, malaise, headache and stiff neck, followed by arthritic pain in the large joints.

Mallory-Weiss tear (lesion)

an esophageal or gastric tear, often due to prolonged or forceful vomiting, as seen in Mallory-Weiss syndrome.

Marfan disease (syndrome)

an autosomal-dominant congenital disorder of collagen and elastic connective tissues characterized by abnormal length of extremities, subluxation of the lens, and cardiovascular abnormalities.

Marie-Bamberger disease

hypertrophic pulmonary osteoarthropathy; a disorder usually affecting the long bones of the arms and legs, often secondary to chronic pulmonary and heart disease.

Marshall-Marchetti-Krantz operation

surgery to relieve stress incontinence where the anterior portion of the urethra, vesical neck, and bladder are sutured to the posterior surface of the pubic bone.

McConckey cocktail

cod liver oil and tomato juice.

Meckel diverticulum

an abnormal sac or pouch near the ileum due to remains of the embryonic yolk sac.

Ménière syndrome (disease)

nausea, vomiting, tinnitus, vertigo and hearing loss caused by disease of the labyrinth.

Millard-Gubler syndrome

Gubler hemiplegia or paralysis; 6th and 7th nerve palsy with contralateral hemiplegia affecting limbs on one side of the body and the face on the other, together with paralysis of outward movement of the eye, caused by infarction of the pons.

Montgomery glands

sweat glands located in the areola of the nipple.

Moore syndrome

abdominal epilepsy; producing paroxysmal abdominal pain as a sign of an abnormal neuronal discharge from the brain.

Moro reflex

startle reflex; contraction of the limb and neck muscles in infants when startled by a sudden noise, jolt or a short drop.

Munchausen syndrome

repeated presentation to a physician and/or hospital with claims of an acute illness that is false, for the purpose of gaining medical attention.

McBurney's point

site in the right lower abdominal quadrant which is the point of maximum pain in appendicitis.

Niemann-Pick disease

sphingolipidosis; autosomal-recessive inherited lipid histiocytosis with accumulation of phospholipid (sphingomyelin) in histiocytes in the liver, spleen, lymph nodes and bone marrow.

Osgood-Schlatter disease

osteochondrosis of the tibial tuberosity as seen in adolescents.

Osler disease

polycythemia vera or erythremia; chronic disease characterized by bone marrow hyperplasia, increase in blood volume as well as in number of red cells, redness of the skin, and splenomegaly.

Paget disease

(1) osteitis deformans; (2) intraductal carcinoma of the breast; (3) neoplasm of the vulva.

Pancoast tumor

adenocarcinoma of the lung involving pain in the shoulder and arm due to 8th cervical and 1st thoracic nerve involvement.

Parkinson disease

paralysis agitans; a neurological disorder characterized a reduction in dopamine levels, hypokinesia, tremors, and muscular rigidity.

Patau syndrome

trisomy 13 syndrome; a chromosomal abnormality in which an extra chromosome 13 causes defects of the central nervous system, mental retardation, with cleft palate, polydactyly and cardiac problems, among others.

Pel-Epstein fever

the cyclic fever common with Hodgkin disease featuring intermittent febrile episodes lasting for several days.

Pepper syndrome

neuroblastoma of the adrenal gland with metastases in the liver.

Pickwickian syndrome

name derived from the overweight boy in Charles Dickens' *Pickwick Papers*; obesity, somnolence and hypoxia with carbon dioxide retention.

Pott fracture

fracture of the lower fibula and injury of the lower tibial articulation, producing outward displacement of the foot.

Prinzmetal angina

angina pectoris in which attacks occur during rest and for longer duration, accompanied by an ST segment elevation.

Raynaud phenomenon

intermittent ischemia of the fingers or toes marked by severe pallor and often accompanied by paralysis or pain, precipitated by exposure to the cold.

Reiter syndrome (disease)

urethritis, arthritis and conjunctivitis, sometimes with diarrhea.

Reye syndrome

rare, often fatal, disease of children following an acute febrile illness such as influenza or varicella infection, characterized by recurrent vomiting, encephalopathy, hepatomegaly and fatty degeneration of the viscera.

Ritter disease

staphylococcal scalded skin syndrome; usually seen in infants where large areas of skin peel off, as in a second-degree burn, as a result of upper respiratory staphylococcal infection.

Rivers cocktail

Philadelphia cocktail; dextrose in saline with thiamine and insulin given intravenously to detoxify alcoholics.

Romberg sign

closing the eyes increases unsteadiness in a standing patient indicating a loss of proprioceptive control.

Roux-en-Y anastomosis (operation)

a Y-shaped anastomosis which includes the small intestine.

Sabin vaccine

live oral attenuated poliovirus vaccine.

Salk vaccine

original poliovirus vaccine containing inactivated strains of the poliomyelitis virus.

Sjögren syndrome

keratoconjunctivitis sicca, xerostomia and rheumatoid arthritis, usually seen in menopausal women.

Skene glands

paraurethral glands; mucous glands located in the wall of the female urethra.

Stein-Leventhal syndrome

polycystic ovary syndrome; sclerocystic disease of the ovaries commonly characterized by hirsutism, obesity, amenorrhea, infertility and enlarged ovaries.

Stevens-Johnson syndrome

severe, sometimes fatal, bullous form of erythema multiforme involving the mucous membranes.

Stokes-Adams syndrome

a condition caused by heart block with sudden attacks of unconsciousness and seizures.

Strümpell-Marie disease

ankylosing or rheumatoid spondylitis; arthritis of the spine resembling rheumatoid arthritis usually affecting young males.

Swan-Ganz catheter

flexible, flow-directed cardiac catheter featuring a balloon tip to measure pressure in the pulmonary artery.

Tay-Sachs disease

cerebral sphingolipidosis, infantile type; amaurotic familial idiocy (obsolete); an inherited disease appearing at 3 to 6 months of age, characterized by doll-like facies, cherry-red macular spot, loss of vision and progressive spastic paralysis.

Tommaselli syndrome (disease)

fever and hematuria due to quinine overdose.

Treacher Collins syndrome

mandibulofacial dysostosis limited to the orbit and malar regions.

Turner sign

discoloration of the groin following acute pancreatitis.

Unna boot

zinc oxide and gelatin paste used to treat varicose ulcers.

Vincent disease (gingivitis)

necrotizing ulcerative gingivitis; trench mouth; characterized by gingival erythema and pain, fetid odor, and necrosis and sloughing giving rise to a gray pseudomembrane.

von Hippel-Lindau disease

hereditary phakomatosis characterized by retinal and cerebral angiomas.

von Recklinghausen disease

neurofibromatosis characterized by café au lait spots, intertriginous freckling, iris hamartomas and other neurofibromas.

von Willebrand disease

hereditary bleeding disorder also known as angiohemophilia or vascular hemophilia; characterized by a deficiency of coagulating Factor VIII with a tendency to bleed from the mucous membranes for a prolonged period of time.

Wenckebach phenomenon

a cardiac arrhythmia where the P-R interval grows progressively longer until a beat is dropped.

Wilks syndrome

myasthenia gravis

Wolff-Parkinson-White syndrome

paroxysmal tachycardia (or atrial fibrillation) and preexcitation in which the electrocardiogram displays a short P-R interval and a wide QRS complex.

Zenker diverticulum

pharyngoesophageal diverticulum; the most common diverticulum at the junction of the esophagus and the pharynx.

Zollinger-Ellison syndrome

multiple endocrine neoplasia featuring peptic ulceration, gastric hyperacidity and pancreatic gastrin-secreting non-beta islet cell tumors.